the
oh she glows
cookbook

MICHAEL JOSEPH

an imprint of

PENGUIN BOOKS

the
oh she glows
cookbook

Over 100 vegan recipes
to glow from the inside out

Angela Liddon

MICHAEL JOSEPH

UK | USA | Canada | Ireland | Australia
India | New Zealand | South Africa

Michael Joseph is part of the Penguin Random House group of companies
whose addresses can be found at global.penguinrandomhouse.com.

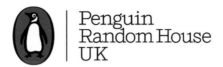

Penguin
Random House
UK

First published in Canada by Penguin Canada Books Inc, 2014
First published in Great Britain by Michael Joseph, 2015
002

Photographs on pages v, x, xviii, 28, 56, 78, 102, 128, 146, 190, 274 and 276
courtesy of Dave Biesse.Photographs on pages 214 and 258 courtesy of Eric Liddon;
all other photographs courtesy of Angela Liddon.

Set in Horley
Printed in China by C&C

A CIP catalogue record for this book is available from the British Library

ISBN: 978–0–71818150–5

www.greenpenguin.co.uk

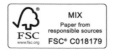

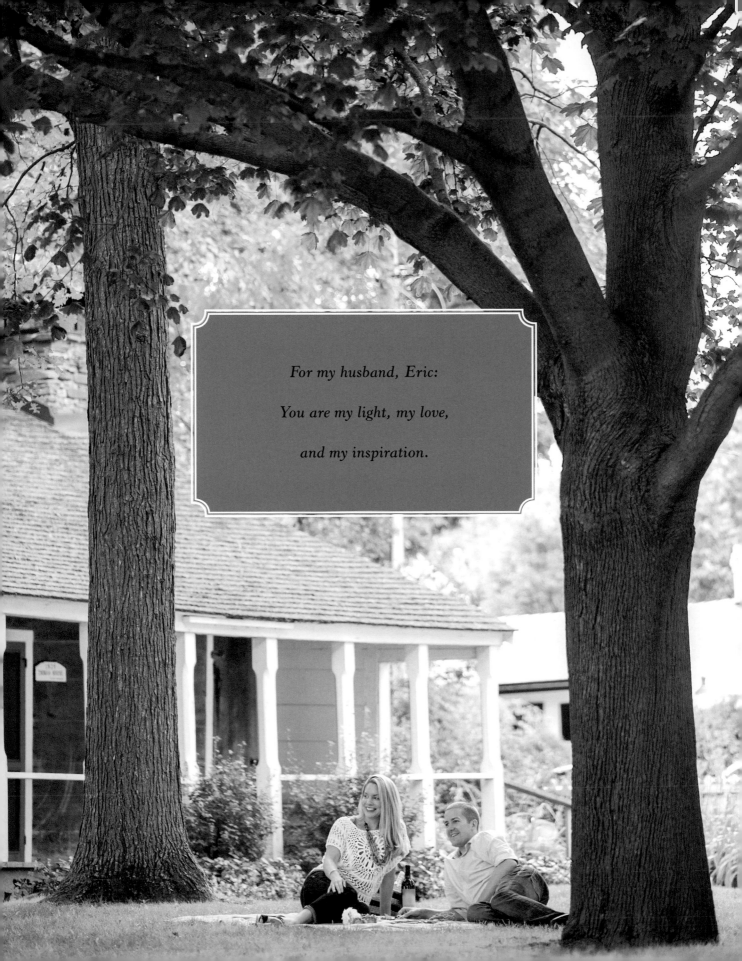

For my husband, Eric:

You are my light, my love,

and my inspiration.

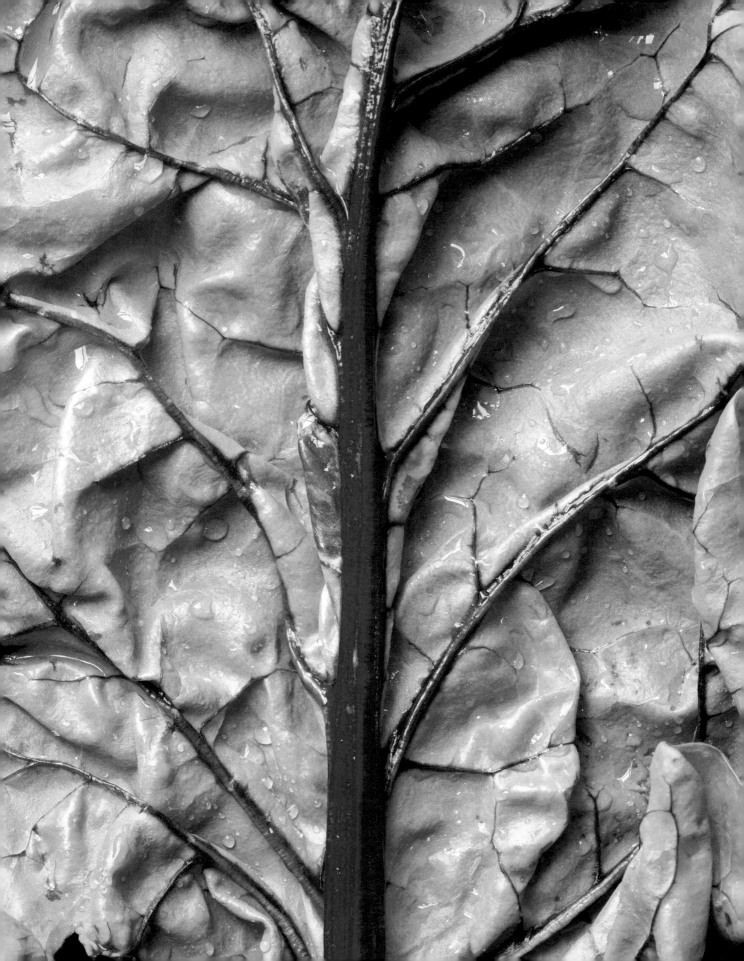

contents

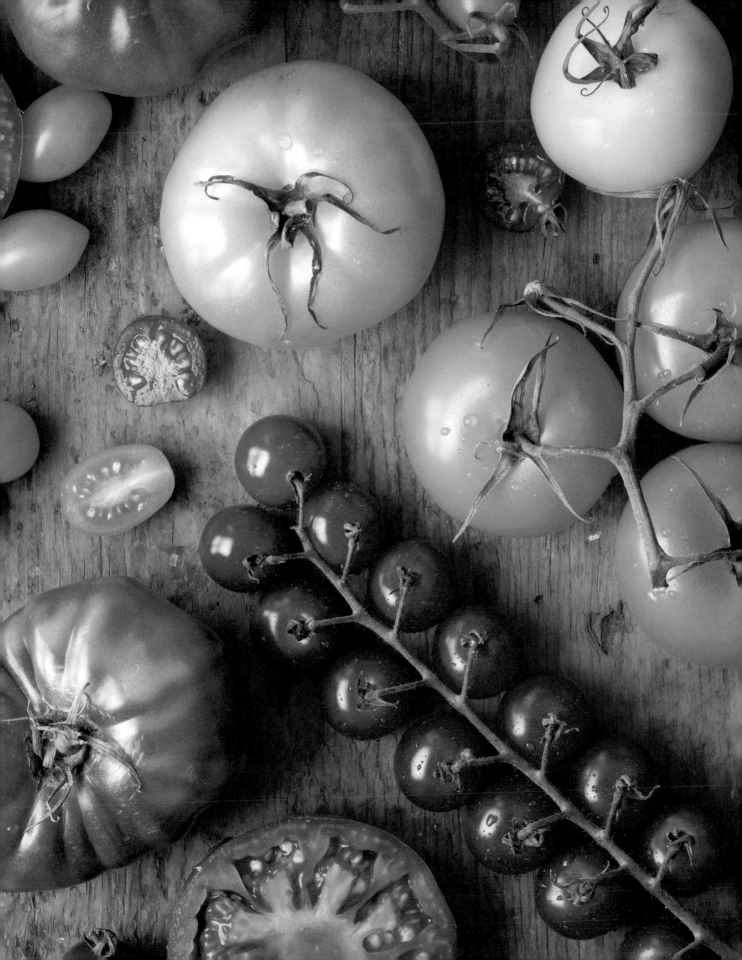

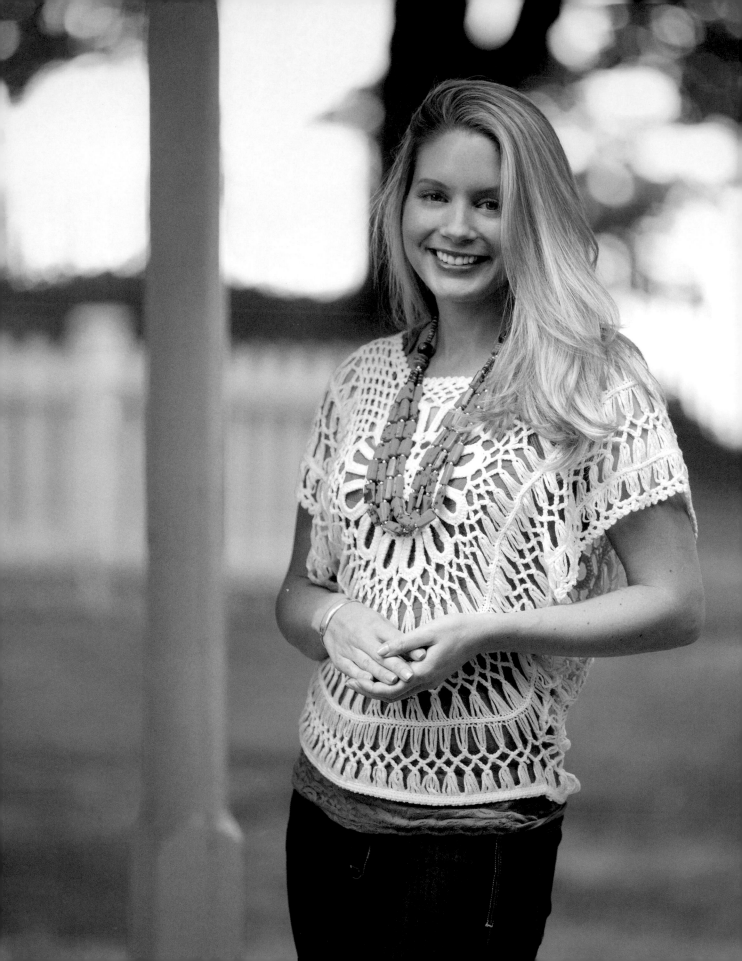

introduction

When I made the switch to a whole foods vegan diet five years ago, I witnessed a powerful transformation in myself. After a decade of struggling with an eating disorder and subsisting on low-calorie, processed, 'diet' foods, I knew I needed to change my life – and my health – for the better. Gradually, I shifted my diet to focus on wholesome plant-based foods, and I was immediately struck by how amazing I felt eating this way. Vibrant vegetables and fruit, whole grains, beans, legumes, nuts, and seeds took the place of highly processed food from a box. Little by little, my skin started to glow, my energy levels soared and my chronic IBS lessened in severity. Those 100-calorie packs of processed cardboard suddenly didn't seem so appealing.

In 2008, I started my blog, *Oh She Glows*, to spread the word about my journey to health and the powerful transformation that food can make in our lives. My goal was, and still is, to share my story openly and to hopefully inspire others who are struggling. To be honest, I didn't know if I would stick with blogging for more than a couple of weeks, but this hobby unexpectedly turned into a full-blown passion, and I can confidently say that my blog changed my entire life. Within the first few months, my readership grew rapidly, and before long, I was connected with readers all over the world. One by one, comments and e-mails sharing stories of pain and triumph started to trickle in. Hearing from courageous women and men became a pivotal tool in my own recovery, as it motivated me to stay on a healthy path. It was the first time in my life that I truly felt fulfilled by the work that I was doing. Before long, I found myself spending countless hours in the kitchen transforming my favorite recipes using plant-based foods, then racing to the computer to share the pictures and recipes with my blog readers.

Five years later, *Oh She Glows* has grown beyond my wildest dreams, receiving millions of page views a month. Over the years, I've heard from readers all over the world who have experienced positive health changes after embracing my recipes. I feel so grateful to be able to share my passion with others, spreading my joy for healthy food around the world. For years, it's been a personal dream to write a cookbook, a place where I could share my most treasured recipes, such as go-to breakfasts, protein-packed snacks, hearty mains and decadent desserts. I am simply delighted to finally share this collection of recipes that I've had to keep secret until now. *The Oh She Glows Cookbook* is packed with more than one hundred recipes that will have you glowing from the inside out, including seventy-five new and exclusive recipes plus a few dozen new-and-improved reader favourites. Whether you are a vegan or you simply want to incorporate a few vegan meals into your week, I'm confident the recipes in this cookbook will have a positive impact on your health and well-being, and hopefully renew your enthusiasm for simple, plant-based eating.

MY JOURNEY TO HEALTH

I wish I could begin my story with a romantic tale about growing up on a farm and learning to cook treasured family recipes from a grandparent. But the truth is my turbulent, on-again, off-again relationship with food has been fraught with challenges. For more than ten years, food was the enemy in my life. I struggled with the two extremes of self-starvation and binge eating, a vicious roller coaster that left me insecure, suspicious of food, and ultimately miserable in my own skin. At the time, I didn't consider how the food I ate each day impacted on the way I felt, nor did I really care. Obsessing over calories and fat grams was indeed a mask for other issues in my life, but it also prevented me from truly appreciating the power of proper nutrition and its ability to impact my mood, my energy levels and even my self-esteem. Deep down, I knew I held the power to create a huge change in my life, but I didn't quite know how to *make* the change.

The truth is that our finest moments are most likely to occur when we are feeling deeply uncomfortable, unhappy, or unfulfilled. For it is only in such moments, propelled by our discomfort, that we are likely to step out of our ruts and start searching for different ways or truer answers. – M. SCOTT PECK

In my twenties, I began the long road of recovery from my eating disorder. With a new sense of optimism, I allowed myself to look beyond the past and embark on a journey of personal healing. My goal was simple: learn to love real food again and eat wholesome foods that made me glow from the inside out. That meant ditching the 100-calorie snacks, artificially sweetened fat-free yogurt and chemical-laden zero-calorie butter spray for good! Instead, I started to blend leafy greens and other vegetables into my morning smoothies before work each day. You name it, I threw it into my blender – from kale and cucumbers to beets and carrots. My first attempts were a bit scary-looking (and -tasting) – hence the name Green Monsters (see pages 57, 59, and 67) – but eventually, I started blending up delicious concoctions and sharing the recipes on my blog. Much to my surprise, Green Monsters took the blog world by storm, and readers from all over the world began sending me pictures of their own Green Monster smoothies. Soon enough, my skin started to get its glow back and I reclaimed the energy I needed to power through my busy days. My husband, Eric, also reaped the rewards of plant-based foods by dropping twenty pounds and reducing his high cholesterol without any medication. These positive results motivated me to stick to this new lifestyle and not fall back into old negative patterns.

Let food be thy medicine and medicine be thy food. – HIPPOCRATES

I started to bring more plants into my kitchen with the help of a Community Supported Agriculture (CSA) vegetable subscription and frequent trips to the farmer's market. A couple of years later, I planted my own vegetable garden and grew oodles of kale and other veggies (I won't tell you about all the herbs I killed, though!). Growing my own vegetable garden was the first time I truly felt connected to the food on my plate. I was simply amazed to see real vegetables growing in my garden, vegetables that

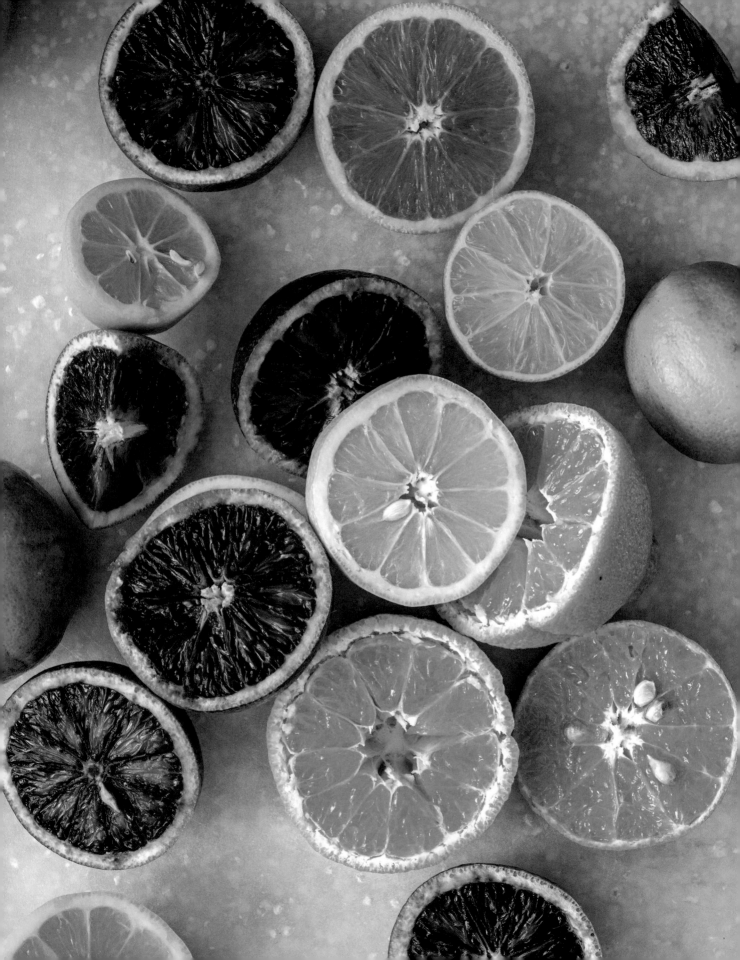

I could pull from the soil and eat! Everything was flavourful and fresh, just like nature intended. For the first time in my life, I got busy in the kitchen, teaching myself how to cook food (and photograph it) from scratch. There were countless cooking disasters (many of which I documented on my blog), but also many successes, and these encouraged me to keep learning and improving my culinary talent.

As I fell in love with real food, I started to experiment with vegan recipes that I found online, but I was often disappointed with the results. Many recipes were hit-and-miss, lacked flavour, and were often highly processed or called for mock meat products. Discouraged by these initial recipe flops, I vowed to create my own reliable vegan recipe collection that could win over even the most devout meat-lover. If my recipes didn't please my husband, they didn't make the cut, so I made it my mission to teach myself how to create drool-worthy meals, often testing recipes multiple times before I shared them on my blog. Best of all, my recipes feature wholesome, plant-based foods that make me feel anything but deprived. Throughout this process, I've realized you don't have to sacrifice flavour, variety, or nutrition to enjoy vegan recipes. When you use fresh ingredients, the food speaks for itself.

My transition to a vegan diet was made up of small and incremental changes; I didn't throw everything out of my fridge one day or declare war on animal products and processed foods with the snap of a finger. It was a gradual process, and because of this it has been a long-lasting and sustainable lifestyle change. Initially, I purchased a lot of fake meat and other vegan products, but I quickly discovered that my energy and overall health fared better when I didn't rely on these products. Because of this, you won't find a lot of imitation vegan foods in this cookbook. My diet is made up primarily of vegetables, fruit, whole grains, nuts, legumes, seeds, and minimally processed soy products, so those are the predominant ingredients you'll find in this cookbook. I used to think that *vegan* was a code word for weird, limited, or unappetizing food, but I've since proved myself wrong. If you are one of those sceptics, I hope to change your mind, too!

As I started to eat fewer animal products and more plants, I felt – and looked – like a new person. Perhaps this was a vain motivation in the beginning, but over time my motivation increased in so many other ways. After learning about the horrors of meat and dairy factory farming, I had to ask myself some hard questions. How could I, the lifelong animal lover, continue to support a system that brought so much pain and suffering to so many animals each year? The complete dichotomy of the food on my plate and my passion for animal welfare was, quite frankly, hard to digest. Wasn't there

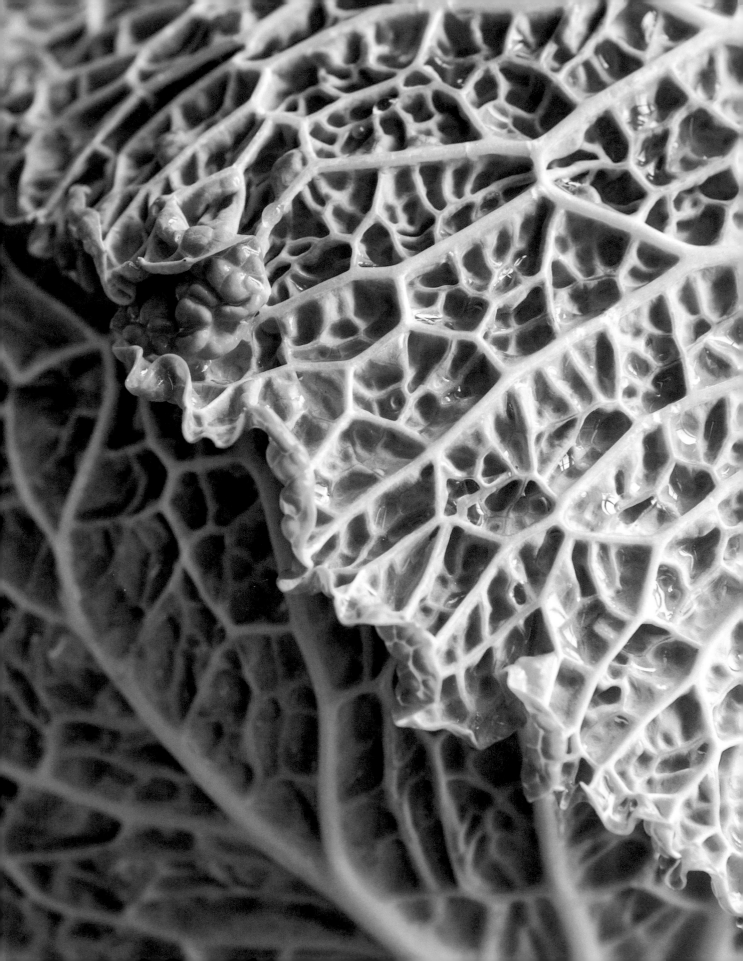

another solution? Couldn't I eat a healthy, well-rounded diet without contributing to a system that I didn't believe in?

Yes, I certainly could. A vegan diet encouraged me to look outward for healing and to value all walks of life, including my own. Little by little, I found the growth that I so desperately needed – through food. A vegan diet is the way I aligned what's in my heart with the food on my plate. My compassion for others – and, most surprising, for myself – grew in many ways. I finally realized that I'm worthy of happiness and deserving of nourishment no matter what the scale says – we all are.

It's my hope that the recipes in this book will not only ignite your culinary fire, but also show you how easily you can incorporate healthy vegan recipes into your own diet. Feeling good starts with what we eat and from there spreads like wildfire to other areas in your life. So go out and chase your long-desired career change, run that 10k, and fall in love with kale. There's no better time than now!

– *Angela*

Never doubt that a small group of thoughtful, committed citizens can change the world. Indeed, it is the only thing that ever has. – Margaret Mead

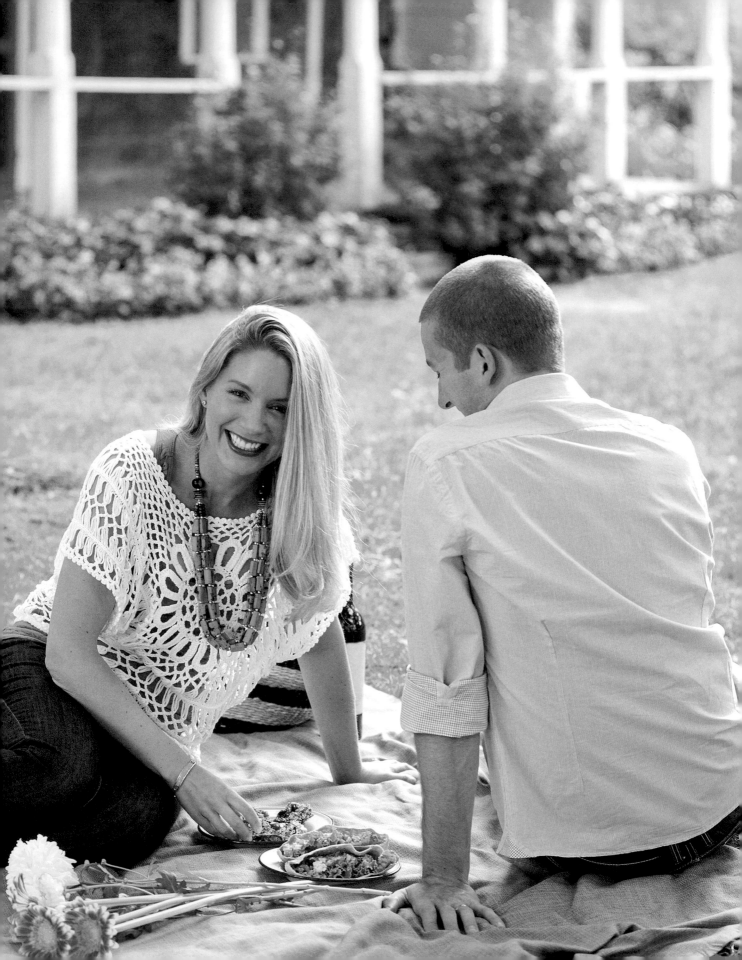

about this book

The Oh She Glows Cookbook is divided into ten different chapters, from Breakfast to Homemade Staples. Many recipes naturally fall into more than one category (for example, the Oil-Free Baked Falafel Bites appetizer also make a satisfying main course (see page 95), so feel free to pick and choose from the various chapters to build your own custom meals.

I encourage you to read the entire headnote and recipe before beginning a recipe. Some recipes require advance preparation (such as soaking nuts), so it helps to plan ahead whenever possible. Most recipes include one or more tips, so be sure to read those, too. Often I'll provide a tip for advance preparation or a way to modify the recipe into something new. For example, my Chilled Chocolate-Espresso Torte can be transformed into freezer fudge very easily (see the Tip on page 242). I've got your back!

I'm aware of how many people are suffering with food allergies or sensitivities these days. Whenever possible, I make a note of possible ingredient substitutions. I'll also let you know if the recipe is gluten-free, refined sugar-free or sugar-free, soy-free, nut-free, grain-free, and/or oil-free, for your convenience. Always be proactive, however, and check the labels of your ingredients to ensure the food is safe for you to consume.

My Natural Foods Pantry (see page 1) details the ingredients that I use most often in my cooking. While it's not intended to encompass every ingredient you might use in your cooking, it does provide a good starting point for the ingredients most frequently used in this cookbook. I recommend reading through this chapter before beginning for an overview of the ingredients and to pick up some tips I've provided about each.

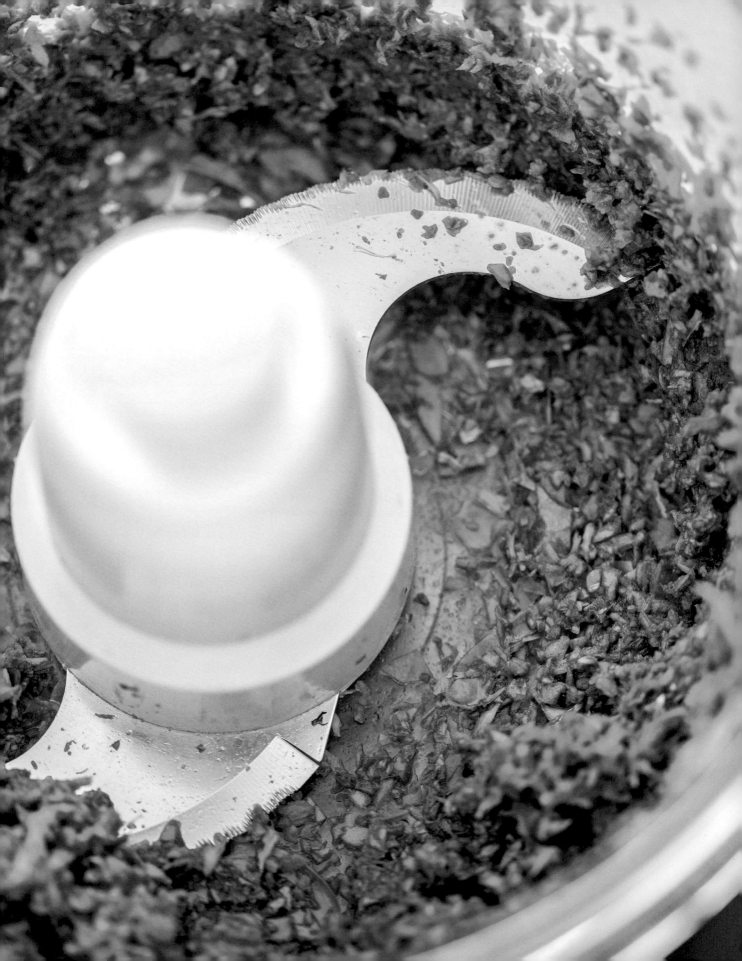

the
oh she glows
cookbook

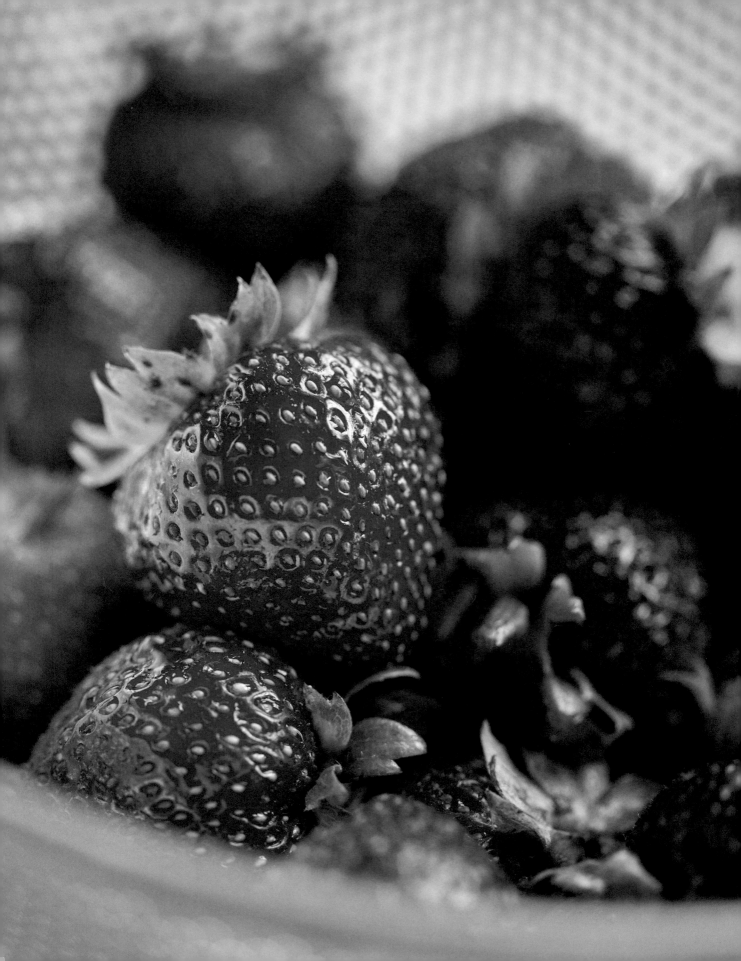

my natural foods pantry

Calling the setup that I have in my kitchen a 'pantry' is amusing to me because when I developed the recipes for this cookbook, we didn't have a pantry or even a decent amount of storage space. (Don't be fooled by the gorgeous 'loaner' kitchen that we used in some of the photographs!) I shoved every ingredient possible into our cupboards, but the overflow often spilled out into our main living area. I hid muffin tins under the coffee table, used the TV cabinet to store bags of flour, and stowed excess pots and pans above the kitchen cabinets. (A girl's gotta do what a girl's gotta do.) Needless to say, it was a bit embarrassing having family and friends over to witness such chaos! My poor husband didn't know what he was signing up for when he proposed; my only saving grace is that he's extremely patient and enjoys his role as Head Taste-Tester Extraordinaire (he made me write that).

Regardless of the setup you have in your own kitchen, stocking the right ingredients makes it so much easier to enjoy a balanced diet. As I learned more about natural, plant-based alternatives to common animal products, I started building a natural foods pantry. It takes time to create, so don't be discouraged if you don't have many of the items just yet. Try adding something new each week and you will be well on your way. Have fun with the journey, above all. And hey, if you have an actual pantry, more power to you!

WHOLE GRAINS & FLOURS

Rolled oats & oat flour

Oats are a great source of fibre and are packed with minerals such as manganese, selenium, phosphorus, magnesium, and zinc. Not only do they provide a lightly sweet, nutty flavour in baked goods, but they can be used in a wide variety of sweet and savoury recipes. Rolled oats (also known as old-fashioned oats) are simply raw oat groats that are steamed and pressed (or rolled) to create their flat shape. Because rolled oats have a large surface area, they cook much more quickly than oat groats and steel-cut oats. Oat flour is incredibly easy to make at home (see page 277) and it adds a rustic, earthy, and lightly sweet quality to baked goods. Be sure to use certified gluten-free oats if you have a gluten allergy or sensitivity, since oats have the potential for cross-contamination with wheat products.

Almond meal & almond flour

Almond meal and almond flour lend a chewy texture and sweet, nutty flavour to cookies, bars, and other baked goods. Almond flour is made from ground blanched (skinless) almonds and has a delicate and fine texture, while almond meal is made from whole almonds (with the skin intact), making it a bit coarser in texture. Almonds are a rich source of protein – 7.6 grams in 35 grams – as well as manganese, vitamin E, magnesium, and copper, making it a healthy flour like no other. You can make almond flour and almond meal in your own kitchen if you have a high-speed blender or food processor (see page 277) or you can find them in most grocery stores in the speciality foods, gluten-free, or organic baking aisles.

100% whole wheat pastry flour

Whole wheat pastry flour is lower in protein and gluten compared to regular whole wheat flour, and its feathery-light texture makes it perfect for replacing traditional all-purpose flour in recipes while retaining more nutrition. I use whole wheat pastry flour to replace some or all of the all-purpose flour called for in recipes like muffins and cakes. A word of caution: Whole wheat pastry flour should not be substituted with 100% whole wheat flour as regular whole wheat flour can produce very dense, heavy baked goods. If you'd like to replace the whole wheat pastry flour with all-purpose flour, however, feel free to do so.

Raw buckwheat groats & raw buckwheat flour

Buckwheat is not a wheat grain like many assume; it's actually a fruit seed related to rhubarb and sorrel. Fortunately, however, buckwheat behaves very similarly to a grain, making buckwheat flour popular for gluten-free baking. Beige and pale green in color, raw buckwheat groats are simply the raw harvested kernels from the plant, and they are a source of protein, fibre, manganese, and magnesium. Kasha, which is toasted buckwheat, is commonly confused with buckwheat groats, but they cannot be used interchangeably in my recipes. Kasha has a much stronger (and some say off-putting) flavour and can throw off the flavour profile of a recipe. For this reason, I always use raw buckwheat groats in my recipes. On page 277, I describe how to make raw buckwheat flour at home. You can find raw buckwheat groats in the bulk bins at many natural grocery stores, such as Whole Foods, or online.

Unbleached all-purpose flour

Unbleached all-purpose flour is made from milled hard and soft wheat and lends a tender, fluffy texture to baked goods. I don't use all-purpose flour in many of my recipes, but sometimes it's the only flour that will produce the light texture required for cake or pastry recipes. Even then, I find it's usually possible to substitute one-third of the all-purpose flour for whole wheat pastry flour without compromising the overall outcome (see my Double-Layer Chocolate Fudge Cake on page 249 for an example). Be sure to look for organic, unbleached varieties of all-purpose flour whenever possible.

In addition to those listed above, I also use brown rice and brown rice flour, wild rice, millet, quinoa, spelt and wheat berries, and brown rice, kamut, or spelt pasta on a regular basis.

NON-DAIRY MILK, YOGHURT & CHEESE

For those looking to ditch dairy, non-dairy milk options are plentiful in most grocery stores these days. My personal favorite non-dairy milk is almond milk. I use it exclusively in my recipes, but feel free to use your preferred non-dairy milk. I make almond milk at home (see page 275) for drinking and I buy unsweetened and unflavoured almond milk for my recipes. Almond milk is very low in protein, so if you want a higher-protein non-dairy milk (say, for smoothies), look for soy milk or hemp milk. I also use canned coconut milk in many of my dessert recipes. It adds a rich, creamy quality very similar to dairy cream. My go-to brands of coconut milk are Native Forest and Thai Kitchen. As for non-dairy yoghurt and cheese, these are not products that I use often, but I do use them once in a while. In my Spa Day Bircher Muesli recipe (page 37), I use non-dairy yoghurt. I prefer the flavour of almond and coconut yoghurt (such as So Delicious brand), but feel free to use soy yoghurt for a higher-protein option. In my Crowd-Pleasing Tex-Mex Casserole (page 149), I use a small amount of vegan shredded cheese. My preferred brand is Daiya, but again, feel free to use your preferred non-dairy cheese.

SWEETENERS

Medjool dates

Soft and plump Medjool dates – is there anything better? I love using Medjool dates as a natural sweetener in smoothies, no-bake desserts, and even pie crusts (see page 247). They aren't called nature's candy for nothing! They're also fantastic for binding ingredients and enhancing flavour with sweet notes of caramel. Just try my Homemade Yolos on page 263 for proof – many say they're better than the store-bought candy! If you don't have Medjool dates on hand, other varieties of dates should work in a pinch. If your dates are firm and dry, be sure to soften them in water for 30 to 60 minutes before using – and, of course, always remove the pit.

100% pure maple syrup

It probably comes as no surprise that this Canadian girl is a huge fan of maple syrup. Maple syrup is simply the boiled sap of maple trees, and it's my sweetener of choice because it is easy to source locally. Look for grade B syrup, which tends to have the most robust flavour. I realize pure maple syrup is not available everywhere and can be expensive depending on your location, so when you can't get your hands on it, feel free to substitute your preferred liquid sweetener, such as agave nectar. The flavour of the recipe will change, but the overall recipe should still turn out fine, as long as you are subbing a liquid sweetener for another liquid sweetener. I don't recommend subbing a liquid sweetener for a dry sweetener because it throws off the wet/dry ratio in a recipe and the outcome is unpredictable.

Sucanat sugar

Sucanat (which stands for Sugar Cane Natural) is a minimally processed organic form of whole cane sugar with a grainy, coarse texture similar to coconut sugar. To make Sucanat, sugarcane juice is extracted from the sugar cane and then heated in a large vat. Once the juice cooks down into thick syrup, it's cooled and dried. This process retains the molasses content, which provides naturally occurring minerals and vitamins (such as iron, calcium, and potassium) in the sugar and provides a caramel hue and robust flavour. I love to use Sucanat in gingerbread or chocolate recipes (see Oil-Free Chocolate-Courgette Muffins, page 227, or Fudgy Mocha Pudding Cake, page 257) or anywhere I'd normally use traditional brown sugar. If you don't have any Sucanat on hand, feel free to substitute unpacked organic brown sugar or coconut sugar in its place.

Coconut sugar

Coconut sugar is coconut palm sap that has been cooked over low heat, cooled, dried, and ground into a granulated sugar. Despite the fact that it comes from a coconut palm tree, it doesn't have a coconut flavour so it blends seamlessly into many recipes while adding light notes of caramel. Not only does it have a low glycemic index (35) compared to other sweeteners, but it is rich in vitamins and minerals. You can substitute coconut sugar for Sucanat or unpacked organic light brown sugar in most recipes.

Organic cane sugar & organic brown sugar

Organic cane sugar is an all-purpose sweetener used in baked goods. It's very similar to traditional white sugar, but organic cane sugar isn't processed with animal bone char, nor is it whitened with bleach! Organic brown sugar is almost identical to cane sugar, only it has a bit of molasses added in, providing its characteristic brown colour as well as a higher moisture content. Feel free to use either light or dark brown sugar in my recipes.

Blackstrap molasses

Blackstrap molasses is a powerhouse sweetener packed with iron, potassium, calcium, magnesium, and more. This thick, robust syrup produces moist and chewy baked goods, and is great in gingerbread, ginger cookies, BBQ sauces, and more. Each tablespoon of blackstrap molasses contains 3.5 milligrams iron, making it an easy way to boost your iron stores. Be sure to pair blackstrap molasses with vitamin C for maximum iron absorption.

Brown rice syrup

Brown rice syrup delivers a steady and consistent energy supply and is said to be good for avoiding blood sugar spikes due to its relatively low glycemic index. I don't use brown rice syrup very often, but I do use it in a couple of my recipes (see my Glo Bar recipes on pages 215 and 217) as a binder thanks to its super-sticky consistency. There have been recent concerns about arsenic levels in brown rice syrup and other rice products, and as a result, research is ongoing to determine safe exposure levels. I encourage you to monitor the research results and make your own informed opinion as to whether to include it in your diet.

FATS/OILS

Virgin coconut oil

Coconut oil is my favourite oil to cook and bake with due to its heart-healthy, antifungal, and antibacterial properties. With its high smoke point, it is also great for high-heat frying, roasting, or grilling without damaging the properties of the oil. For this reason, I use coconut oil more than any other oil in my kitchen. Solid at room temperature, it also makes a great replacement for butter in many recipes and helps raw recipes maintain a solid texture (see my Chilled Chocolate-Espresso Torte, page 241). Virgin coconut oil does taste like coconut and can infuse a light coconut flavour into foods, but I find it's minimal and often complements the recipe. I've grown to love the flavour, so I use it with abandon even when making savoury meals like stir-fries. If you aren't a fan of the flavour of coconut oil, you can try refined coconut oil, which does not have a coconut flavour. In savoury preparations, such as when pan-frying or sautéing, you can easily replace the coconut oil for your preferred cooking oil, if desired.

Cold-pressed extra-virgin olive oil

Extra-virgin olive oil has its place in every kitchen, but it's not to be used for high-heat cooking like frying. Its smoke point of 200°C (400°F) makes it easy to render this delicate oil rancid by using too much heat. Despite this, it's a good all-purpose oil so long as you are careful not to overheat it. When selecting extra-virgin olive oil, look for brands packaged in a dark-amber glass bottle, which blocks out unwanted UV light. Cold-pressed olive oil uses a chemical-free pressure method of extracting the oil, so it's usually considered the healthiest option.

Grapeseed oil

Grapeseed oil is a neutral cooking oil that blends seamlessly into many recipes. I like to use grapeseed oil in cake recipes when I don't want the oil to impact the overall flavour of the cake. Extra-virgin olive oil can also be swapped in for grapeseed oil (except when frying or roasting at high temperatures), but keep in mind that the flavour of the olive oil may come through in the recipe.

Avocado

Have you ever tried using avocado as a butter or oil replacement? It's downright dreamy. Avocado is what they call nature's butter, after all. I love to mash avocado on toast instead of butter (see Sunrise Scramble on page 33) and I also use it as an oil and cream replacement in my Creamy Avocado Pasta recipe (see page 173). Really, what can't avocados do?

Vegan butter

Vegan butter, made from plant-based oil, is everywhere these days, and there are soy-free and palm oil-free varieties becoming available now, too. I use coconut oil more often for its health benefits, but when I feel that a buttery flavour is crucial in a recipe I'll use vegan butter – in small quantities, of course. For example, my Cauliflower Mashed Potato recipe (see page 207) and my Gluten-Free Chocolate-Almond Brownies (see page 259) are enhanced with a small amount of vegan butter, which provides a traditional flavour. Vegan butter is also great spread on muffins, quick breads, baked potatoes, and toast.

Toasted sesame oil & flaxseed oil

In salad dressings, I use flaxseed oil for its rich omega-3 fatty-acid profile and occasionally use toasted sesame oil. Both of these oils have a low smoke point, so it's important not to heat them very much, if at all. See my Effortless Anytime Balsamic Vinaigrette made with flaxseed oil on page 283 and my Thai Peanut Sauce made with toasted sesame oil on page 153. If you don't have either of these oils on hand, feel free to replace them with extra-virgin olive oil.

SALT

Because individual salt preferences vary, I tend to ask you to add salt 'to taste' in my recipes (except in my baked dessert recipes). Use my amount as a general guideline, but trust your own taste buds above all. You can always add more salt, but it's difficult to fix a recipe once you've added too much.

Herbamare

Herbamare is a fantastic herbed salt brand infused with vegetables and herbs like celery, leek, onion, parsley, garlic, basil, rosemary, and more. It's also slightly lower in sodium than traditional table salt, and due to its great flavour I use it liberally when seasoning vegetables. Whenever I'm roasting or sautéing vegetables, you can assume I'm using Herbamare.

Fine-grain sea salt

My go-to all-purpose salt is iodized fine-grain sea salt. Sea salt is made from evaporated saltwater lake or ocean water and retains some trace minerals. Table salt, on the other hand, is mined from underground salt deposits and is heavily processed and often includes additives. I prefer to buy iodized sea salt because iodine is a critical nutrient for healthy thyroid function, and salt is an easy way to obtain this mineral in my diet. I also use pink Himalayan salt, too, when I have it on hand.

Flaked sea salt

Flaked sea salt is certainly not a necessary ingredient, but it's lovely as a finishing element. A little sprinkle on top of brownies or homemade chocolate goes a long way and helps the sweet flavours pop!

HERBS & SPICES

I use the following dried herbs and spices most often:

Cayenne pepper
Chilli powder
Cinnamon
Coriander
Cumin
Garlic powder
Ginger
Onion powder
Oregano
Paprika
Red pepper flakes
Smoked paprika (both sweet and hot varieties)
Turmeric

In general, I try to purchase dried herbs in small quantities from grocery-store bulk bins or bulk-food stores. It's much cheaper to buy loose dried herbs as opposed to paying for those tiny overpriced jars. Contrary to popular belief, dried herbs do not have a very long shelf life and should be replaced often. As a rule of thumb, powdered dried herbs should be replaced every 6 months. Store dried herbs in glass jars in a cool, dark place away from all heat sources (such as the oven). I tend to always use fresh basil, parsley, rosemary, and freshly grated nutmeg in my recipes because I find their flavour is superior when fresh. Fresh ginger is also fantastic in many recipes and has many health benefits, such as improved digestion and immunity (see my Healing Rooibos Tea, page 69, for example).

VEGETABLE BROTH/ BOUILLON POWDER

To save money, I make vegetable broth by mixing boiling water and vegetable bouillon powder. My go-to brand is Go BIO, which is vegan and free of yeast and MSG. Feel free to use homemade vegetable broth (see page 299) or store-bought broth, too.

NUTS/SEEDS

Chia seeds

Bursting with omega-3 fatty acids, iron, calcium, magnesium, fibre, and protein, chia seeds are nutritional powerhouses. I add a tablespoon to my daily smoothies, and I also enjoy tossing chia seeds into my Glo Bars (see pages 215 and 217), baked goods, Effort- less Vegan Overnight Oats (see page 29) and Super-Power Chia Bread (see page 229), or using them as a base for pudding (see Mighty Chia Pudding Parfait on page 225). To keep chia seeds within arm's reach, try filling a salt shaker with chia seeds and placing it on the dinner table. A sprinkle here and a sprinkle there, and you are on your way to a regular consumption of omega-3 fatty acids. Unlike flaxseed, chia seeds do not have to be ground for the nutrients to be absorbed, making them a convenient, fuss-free option. Chia seeds are available online, in bulk food stores and at natural grocers.

Sunflower seeds (shelled)

Vitamin E-rich sunflower seeds are a great seed to have on hand, especially if you have to avoid nuts. If you can't use peanut or almond butter in recipes, sunflower seed butter can be a great alternative. Sunbutter is my go-to brand.

Cashews

Raw cashews are a dairy-free maven's secret weapon. You can create luxurious creamy pies (see Raw Pumpkin-Maple Pie on page 247), homemade dairy-free sour cream (see page 281), cream-based soups (see 10-Spice Vegetable Soup on page 137), and so much more. Once you unlock the power of raw cashews, regular dairy cream will be a distant memory. For many recipes, such as my Cream of Tomato Soup (see page 141), the cashews need to be soaked before use. This makes the cashews softer for ease of blending, and it also makes the nuts easier to digest. To do this, place the cashews in a bowl and add enough water to cover. Soak the cashews for at least 3 to 4 hours, but preferably overnight. Drain and rinse them before using.

Almonds

Raw almonds are packed with calcium, protein and fibre. Just one 35 gram serving of almonds contains 91 milligrams calcium, 7.6 grams protein, and 4 grams fibre, making almonds one of my favorite portable snacks. Like other nuts, the nutrients in almonds are best absorbed when they are soaked in water overnight (otherwise known as 'sprouting') before they are consumed. I like to soak 85 grams of mixed almonds, sunflower seeds, and pepita seeds in a bowl of water overnight (or for about 8 hours). Then I simply drain and rinse them in the morning and place the drained mixture in the fridge for easy grab-and-go snacks. Stored in an airtight container in the refrigerator, they will generally keep for 2 to 3 days.

Flaxseed

Like chia seeds, flaxseed is rich in anti-inflammatory omega-3 fatty acids. Because flaxseed can oxidize quickly, I like to store whole flaxseed in the fridge or freezer and grind just the amount I need right before using – you can grind flaxseed in a blender or coffee grinder very easily. A mixture of ground flaxseed and water also makes a low-

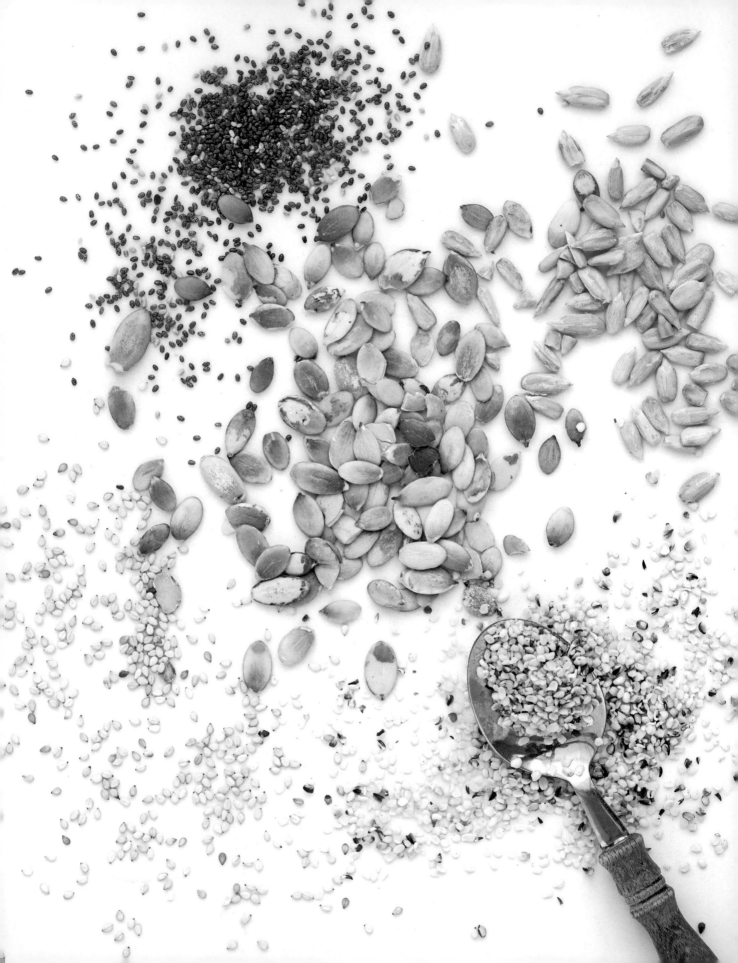

cost egg replacement known as a 'flax egg.' When you mix ground flaxseed with water and let the mixture sit for a few minutes, it thickens and forms a gel-like texture very similar to an egg white.

Hemp seeds (hulled)

Hulled hemp seeds (also called hemp hearts) are soft, tiny green seeds bursting with protein. A complete protein, hemp contains all of the essential amino acids that the human body requires. Three tablespoons contain a whopping 10 grams protein, so you'll be flexing those buff muscles in no time. Even better, hemp seed contains an ideal ratio of omega-6 fatty acids to omega-3 fatty acids (4:1), which helps reduce inflammation in the body. I like to add hemp seeds into smoothies, sprinkle them on salads and oatmeal, and even make hemp-based pesto (see Sun-dried Tomato Kale-Hemp Pesto, page 169).

Pepita seeds (or shelled pumpkin seeds)

Pepita seeds are a great source of protein and iron in any diet. In just 30 grams, pepita seeds pack in almost 10 grams protein and almost 3 milligrams iron. Be sure to pair pepita seeds with vitamin C to maximize iron absorption whenever possible.

To prevent nuts and seeds from becoming rancid, store them in the fridge or freezer. If this isn't possible, store nuts and seeds in a cool, dark place and replenish your stock on a regular basis. In addition to those listed below, I also use unsweetened shredded coconut, sesame seeds (and tahini, a sesame seed paste), roasted all-natural peanut butter, raw pecans, and raw walnuts in my recipes.

BEANS & LEGUMES

Chickpeas (garbanzo beans)

Chickpeas are high in protein, fibre, and iron and 165 grams of cooked chickpeas contains 14.5 grams protein, 12.5 grams fibre, and almost 5 milligrams iron. I rarely go a day without chickpeas – usually in the form of hummus, of course! Bring a fresh batch of hummus over to my house, and we'll be best friends for life (a recipe for Classic Hummus can be found on page 89).

Black beans

With about 15 grams protein and fibre per 172 gram serving, black beans will fill you up and keep hunger at bay. Also known as black turtle beans, these small shiny beans have a dense texture that works well in many vegan dishes like burritos, casseroles (see my Crowd-Pleasing Tex-Mex Casserole, page 149), soups, and salads.

Lentils

Lentils are one of my all-time favorite protein sources, and I cook with them a lot. Not only is Canada the world's largest producer of lentils, but they are incredibly cheap, especially when bought in bulk. Unlike beans, they don't require soaking and can be cooked in 25 to 30 minutes, which make them a great last-minute addition to any meal. Green and brown lentils are the most common, all-purpose lentil varieties and often the easiest to find. They hold their shape quite well if not overcooked and work nicely in a variety of dishes. Red lentils are best in soups and stews because they break down when cooked and help to thicken the broth. French (or Puy) lentils are tiny dark brown or green lentils about half the size of regular green or brown lentils. They hold their shape very well and their chewy texture is a nice addition to fresh salads and pastas. Just 190g of cooked lentils packs in around 18 grams protein, 16 grams fibre, and 6.5 milligrams iron.

A note on soaking and cooking beans:

Before cooking dry beans, it's important to soak them in a large bowl of water for at least 8 to 12 hours prior to cooking. Soaking dry beans before cooking is beneficial in many ways, such as reducing cooking time, improving digestibility, and increasing the availability of minerals.

After soaking, be sure to rinse and drain the beans well before cooking. Get rid of the soaking water – it contains phytates, tannins, and other flatulence-causing substances that have been released by the beans.

To cook the beans, place them in a large saucepan with enough water to cover them by 2.5cm. I also like to add a thumb-size piece of kombu (a type of seaweed) to the pot, as it helps with digestion and also releases beneficial minerals into the cooking water. Bring the water to a boil, then reduce the heat to medium to maintain a simmer. Scoop off and discard any foam that rises to the surface while the beans simmer. Cook for 40 to 60 minutes (depending on the type of bean and its freshness), until the beans are soft and can be pierced with a fork without any resistance.

It's important not to add any salt until after the beans have finished cooking. If you add salt during the cooking process, the beans may not cook evenly; they might be soft in some places and tough in others.

A note on canned goods:
As much as possible, I try to prepare food from scratch, but as we all know, life gets busy! When I need a meal in a pinch, I have no problem using Bisphenol-A (BPA)-free cans. Eden Foods is my go-to brand for canned beans. I typically have their canned chickpeas and black beans, and a jar of their crushed tomatoes on hand at all times. As for BPA-free diced or whole peeled canned tomatoes, I use Ontario Natural brand – made locally and certified organic.

SOY PRODUCTS

Firm or extra-firm organic tofu
I don't use a lot of tofu in my recipes, but when I do, it's always a firm or extra-firm variety because I prefer the texture of firm tofu. Look for organic, non-GMO tofu and other soy products whenever possible.

A note on pressing tofu:
Pressing tofu squeezes out the water for a firmer, denser end result. After a couple of years of pressing my tofu under cookbooks, I finally purchased a tofu press. It's life-changing! If you consume tofu frequently, I highly recommend investing in a tofu press. The ease and convenience are well worth it. If you don't have a tofu press, have no fear. You can press tofu without one (see page 285 for more info).

Edamame
Edamame is a fancy-sounding name for green soybeans. They are sold fresh or frozen

in grocery stores; the frozen variety has usually been pre-boiled or -steamed. Edamame is a great option if you are looking for a quick-cooking complete protein source to add into plant-based meals. I love to use edamame in salads, stir-fries, and dips.

Tempeh

Tempeh is a fermented soy product with a nutty and slightly bitter flavour, the latter of which can be improved by steaming or other cooking methods. It is most commonly sold in the refrigerator section of the grocery store, but it can be found in the freezer section occasionally, too. Its cake-like, rectangular shape is rough and bumpy compared to smooth and soft tofu blocks. Unlike tofu, tempeh doesn't have to be pressed before use due to its low water content. Don't be alarmed if your tempeh block is speckled with white spots or even a bit of black veining (both normal results of the fermentation process), but beware if you see any pink, blue, or yellow colouration. This likely means that the tempeh has gone bad. I'm a late bloomer when it comes to enjoying the wonders of tempeh, but I've shared my all-time favourite tempeh recipe in this book (see Marinated Balsamic, Maple & Garlic Tempeh on page 199). Dare I say it's life-changing? I hope it will make a believer out of you, too!

Wheat-free tamari

Tamari is a type of soy sauce, and it is often gluten-free. I find it to be less salty than traditional soy sauce with a more complex, sweet flavour. Be sure to check the label for certified gluten-free tamari if you are avoiding gluten. Also, look for organic, additive-free tamari to ensure that it's free of artificial colours and flavours. If you need a soy-free alternative, look for coconut aminos, which is similar in flavour and free of soy. Another option is to purchase soy-free tamari, such as by South River brand. I usually buy reduced-sodium tamari to help keep my sodium intake in check.

CHOCOLATE

Dark chocolate chips

It's a rare occurrence when my pantry is out of dark chocolate in some form or another. Not all dark chocolate chips are vegan, but many are. Be sure to read the label carefully to make sure they were not made with any dairy products. Enjoy Life is the brand I purchase the most; their chocolate chips are free of soy, nuts, gluten, and dairy, and they come in mini chocolate chips, the variety I use the most.

Natural unsweetened cocoa powder

Made from roasted cocoa beans, natural (non-alkalized) unsweetened cocoa powder has a bitter taste and lends a rich, deep chocolate flavour to baked goods. It's highly acidic, so when you combine it with baking soda (which is alkaline), it produces a reaction that causes baked goods to rise and expand. Natural cocoa powder is not to be confused with Dutch-process cocoa powder, which is a type of cocoa powder that has been treated with an alkalizing agent. This gives Dutch-processed cocoa powder a milder taste, but it does not produce the same reaction when paired with baking soda. As a result, they are not to be used interchangeably in recipes. I use natural unsweetened cocoa powder throughout this cookbook.

OTHER

Nutritional yeast

Nutritional yeast lends a cheesy, nutty flavour to vegan recipes and is rich in protein and often fortified with B vitamins. It's an inactive, dead form of yeast and is not to be confused with brewer's yeast, which is used to make bread rise. Try nutritional yeast in sauces, gravies, dressings, and sprinkled on popcorn and garlic bread, or make my Life-Affirming Warm Nacho Dip (see page 83) to really knock your socks off.

Baking soda & aluminium-free baking powder

Not only does aluminium-free baking powder taste better (no metallic aftertaste), but it's good to know I'm not putting unwanted aluminium into my body. To test if your baking powder is active, mix ½ teaspoon into 75ml boiling water. If it bubbles, it's active. Baking powder has a shelf life of 6 to 12 months. Baking soda, on the other hand, does not contain aluminium so it's generally safe to buy any brand. To test if baking soda is active, mix ½ teaspoon with some vinegar. If it foams and bubbles, it's active. Baking soda has a very long shelf life of at least 3 years.

Arrowroot powder

Arrowroot powder is a fine, starchy white powder derived from the rootstock of the tropical arrowroot plant. It works well as a thickener in sauces and gravies and it also has binding properties that help ensure successful gluten-free baked goods. If you don't have arrowroot powder on hand, feel free to substitute cornstarch.

Dried kombu

A type of seaweed, kombu is said to aid digestion, helping to break down gas-causing enzymes in beans while cooking. It also infuses food with natural minerals present in the seaweed. I like to add a thumb-size piece of kombu when cooking beans, grains, and legumes from scratch.

ACIDS

Acidic ingredients such as citrus and vinegars add a lovely brightness to dishes and prevent the dish from falling flat in the flavour department. The most common acids I cook with include fresh lemon juice, apple cider vinegar, balsamic vinegar, rice vinegar, red or white wine vinegar, and white vinegar. I try to keep all of these vinegars stocked in my pantry. Due to its acidic nature, vinegar has a very long shelf life and can be stored at room temperature.

my favourite kitchen tools & equipment

Here are the kitchen tools I rely on the most to get the job done. Not all of the items listed below are absolute necessities, but many of them make my life easier each and every day.

FOOD PROCESSOR

I have a 3.5l Cuisinart food processor and use it at least once a day, with all the recipe testing I do. For everyday use, however, you can get away with a smaller version. I use my processor to make energy bites, raw desserts, nut butters, sauces, pesto, and more. I recommend using a heavy-duty processor when making things like nut butter (see my Crunchy Maple-Cinnamon Roasted Almond Butter, page 295) to avoid motor burnout. The smaller machines often can't handle the processing time that's required.

HIGH-SPEED BLENDER

After going through a few blenders early in my journey to health, I said enough is enough and invested in a Vitamix 5200. It's an expensive machine, but totally worth the investment. Another trusted brand is Blendtec; the two are very comparable in terms of quality and blending capability. I use my blender every single day for making smoothies, juices, homemade sauces, soups, homemade almond milk, and home-ground flours. If you don't have a Vitamix, fear not – most high-speed blenders will work in a pinch. Just be aware that some blenders may not blend vegetables like kale or fruit like dates as smooth as you'd like.

GLASS CANNING JARS

Admittedly, I don't do much canning, but I love to use glass canning jars as storage containers in my pantry and fridge. They also make fun drinking glasses for smoothies (see pages 57 to 67). I own a variety of sizes, from about 125ml all the way up to 2l. Just like shoes, you can never have too many glass jars (just don't try to tell my husband that)!

CHEF'S KNIFE & PARING KNIFE

I really didn't know how much easier chopping vegetables could be until I acquired my first good-quality chef's knife. A high-quality chef's knife will easily slice through vegetables without much pressure. Use a chef's knife for all of your general chopping and dicing purposes. A paring knife is excellent for intricate cutting jobs like trimming the rind off an orange or seeding peppers. Be sure to invest in a knife sharpener. Keeping your knives sharp means keeping yourself safe, so make it a habit to sharpen them on a regular basis – plus, you'll kind of feel a bit like Zorro when you do.

MICROPLANE RASP GRATER

This handheld fine grater allows you to zest citrus with finesse and shave chocolate like a pro. Sure, you can also use a box grater, but the Microplane grater is easier to control for all of those small jobs. I like to impress dinner guests with it, too; dazzle them at the table by simply grating a little chocolate on top of their dessert!

LARGE RIMMED BAKING SHEETS

Rimmed baking sheets are perfect for roasting vegetables and chickpeas because the rim prevents anything from falling onto the floor of your oven and burning. If you loathe cleaning your oven like I do, you'll be thankful for this type of pan. Look for the largest size that will fit your oven so you can pack in those vegetables! I purchase eco-friendly baking sheets like Green Pans, which are made without common chemicals like PFOAs (perfluorooctanoic acids).

ENAMELLED DUTCH OVEN

Another investment piece, an enamelled Dutch oven is not cheap, but it will last a lifetime (and beyond) if taken care of properly. Enamelled cast-iron Dutch ovens have a non-toxic, non-stick coating that distributes heat evenly. You can use one on the stovetop or in the oven, making it a convenient all-purpose piece. Since they tend to last for ever, keep your eyes peeled for secondhand pieces at garage sales and antiques markets.

CAST-IRON FRYING PAN

A 25 to 30cm cast-iron frying pan is one of my go-to kitchen tools for a number of reasons. First, while they are a bit more pricey than non-stick ones, you won't have to replace them if you take care of them properly. Second, cooking with cast-iron pans releases trace amounts of iron into your food when cooking, which can be a great thing for vegetarians and vegans. Last, they distribute heat evenly and work well on the stovetop or in the oven.

Be sure to season your pan before use, if necessary. If your pan did not come pre-seasoned, lightly coat the bottom of the pan in oil and bake it in the oven for about 1 hour at 180°C (350°F). After baking, lightly wipe away the excess oil with a paper towel and voilà – the pan is now ready for use. Each time you cook with oil in your cast-iron frying pan, you will build up a natural non-stick coating. A well-seasoned cast-iron pan will eventually become non-stick and require little to no additional oil. To clean your pan, rinse it in hot water immediately after using. It's best not to use soap on

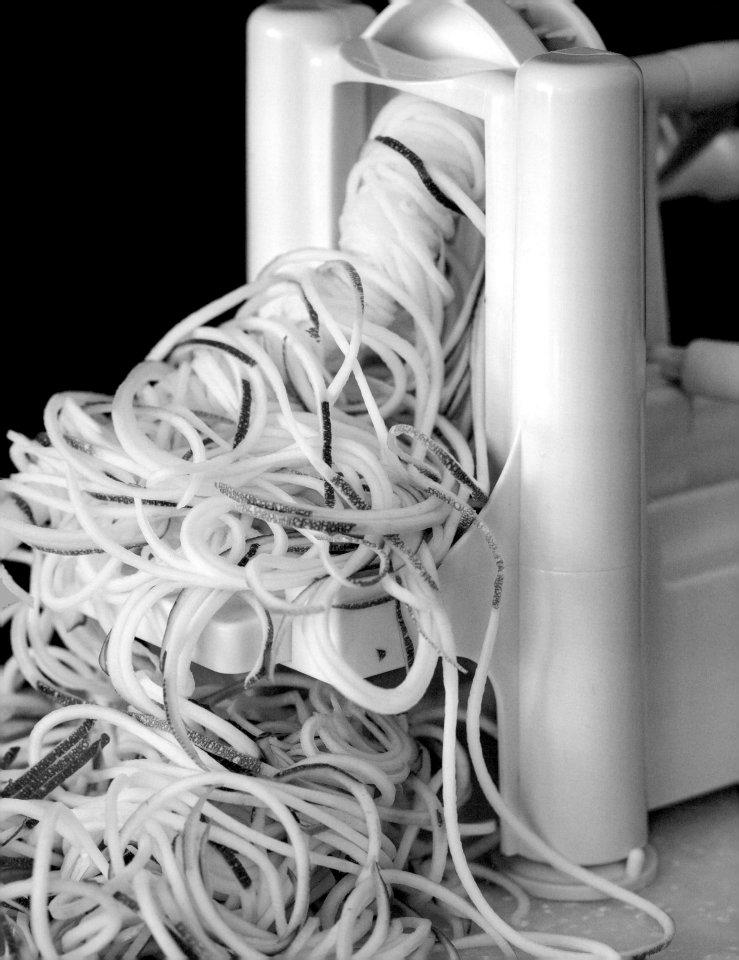

cast-iron pans. If there is food stuck on it, scrub it gently with a non-metal brush and pat it dry with paper towel or an old tea towel (preferably dark in colour, as it can stain linens).

MINI FOOD PROCESSOR

A mini food processor is certainly not a necessity in the kitchen, but I love the compact size for small jobs like making salad dressings or mincing several cloves of garlic in a hurry.

JULIENNE PEELER OR VEGETABLE SPIRALIZER

A julienne peeler is a great tool if you want to thinly slice vegetables like courgette or carrots. My favourite julienne peeler is by Zyliss and costs less than £7. After getting so much use out of my julienne peeler, I upgraded to a vegetable spiralizer, a small, hand-operated appliance used for transforming vegetables like courgette into spaghetti noodles or ribbonlike strands. I use it mainly for courgette in the summer when I want to make a raw pasta dish (see my Immunity-Boosting Tomato Sauce with Mushrooms, page 161). It's a great way to enjoy raw, lighter meals in the summertime without the need for grain-based pasta.

PASTRY ROLLER

A pastry roller is a small roller (usually only around 12cm wide with a short handle. I use it when making my Glo Bars (see pages 215 and 217) or any other time I need to roll out or compress a small area of dough and a rolling pin is too big for the job.

SPRING-RELEASE ICE CREAM SCOOP

Whenever I'm portioning batter into a muffin tin or scooping cookie dough, I use my 30ml stainless-steel ice cream scoop. Look for one that has a spring release because it helps push the batter or dough out without having to fuss with it.

STAINLESS-STEEL WHISK

A stainless-steel whisk is an essential tool in my kitchen. It makes emulsifying wet ingredients by hand a breeze while removing any clumps of flour that most wooden spoons can't break down. I do love my wooden spoons, but sometimes you just need the flick of a whisk!

NUT MILK BAG

My life changed when I purchased my first nut milk bag and started making my own homemade almond milk (see page 275). A nut milk bag is a nylon mesh bag made for straining pulp out of homemade milk or juice. It's reusable (just rinse it immediately after using) and strains blended liquids finer than regular cheesecloth. If you don't want to purchase a nut milk bag, some people have luck using cheesecloth placed over a fine-mesh sieve.

FINE-MESH STAINLESS-STEEL SIEVE

A fine sieve is a small-mesh strainer that works well for several uses. I use mine to rinse small grains like quinoa or millet before use. I also use it to sift flour, cocoa powder, or icing sugar. Last, it can be used to strain homemade juices (see page 71) if you are looking for a smoother texture.

breakfast

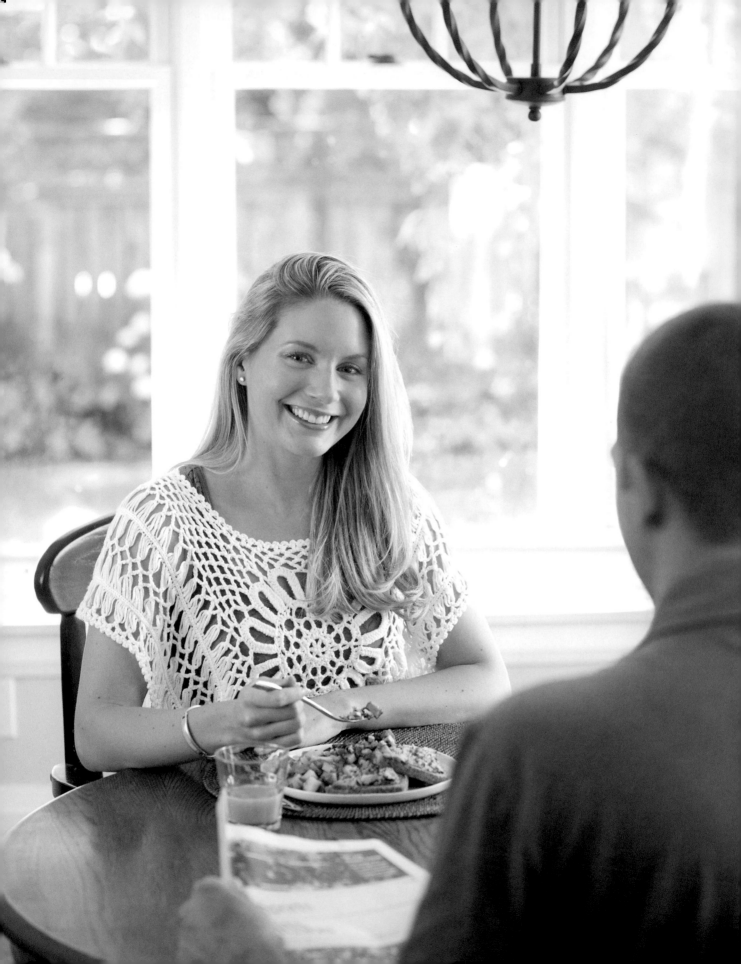

If I had written this book five years ago, this breakfast chapter wouldn't even exist. That's because I spent a good part of my life either skipping breakfast altogether or getting by on a few bites of food. Thankfully – for this book's sake and mine – those days are long behind me! Once I started making healthy breakfasts a part of my daily routine, there was no turning back. Not only do I have more energy and productivity throughout the day, but I enjoy looking forward to a tasty meal when I wake up. Let's face it – being hungry all morning long just isn't fun! In the spring and summer, I tend to crave lighter foods like smoothies (see chapter 2), Effortless Vegan Overnight Oats (page 29), and Raw Buckwheat Breakfast Porridge (page 45), while during cooler months I prefer warming breakfasts such as my Apple Pie Oatmeal (page 49). If you enjoy savoury recipes in the morning, be sure to check out my Loaded Savoury Oatmeal (page 47), Sunrise Scramble (page 33), and Crunchy Seed & Oat Flatbread (page 51). For a holiday brunch or special weekend breakfast, the Maple-Cinnamon Apple & Pear Baked Oatmeal (page 39) never fails to impress a hungry crowd!

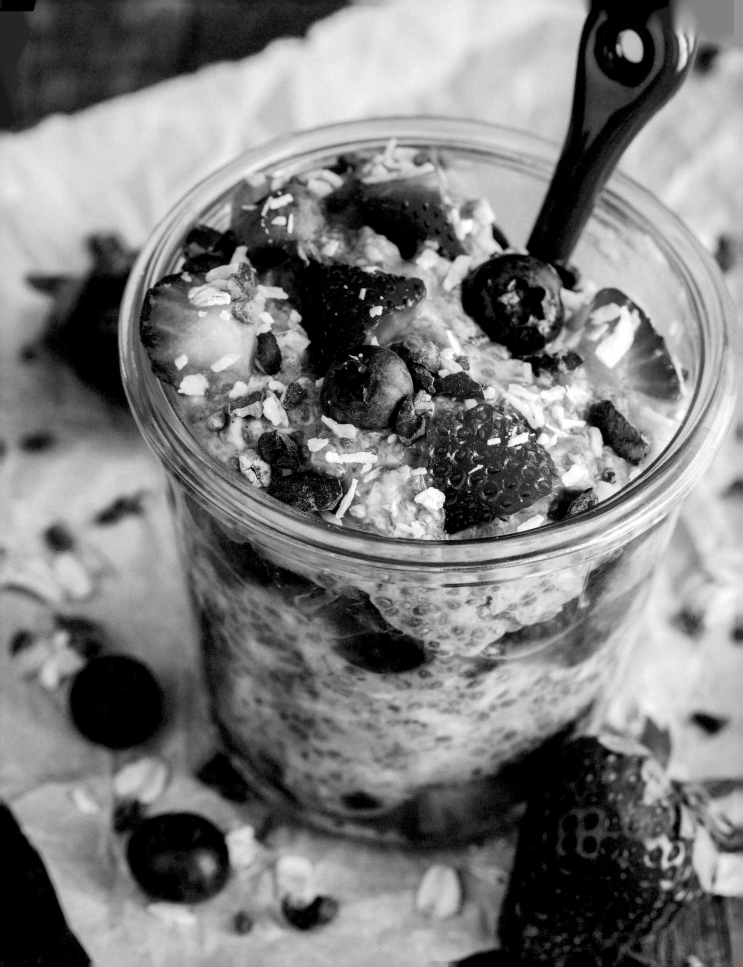

effortless vegan overnight oats

100g gluten-free rolled oats

375ml almond milk

15g chia seeds

1 large banana, mashed

½ teaspoon ground cinnamon

FOR SERVING:
Fresh mixed berries, or other fruit

Ultimate Nutty Granola Clusters (see page 31)

Hemp seeds

Pure maple syrup or other sweetener (optional)

Tips: If your Vegan Overnight Oats have a runny consistency even after they soak, simply stir in an additional 1 tablespoon chia seeds and place the mixture back in the fridge until it has thickened up. If the oat mixture is too thick, simply add a splash of milk and stir to combine.

   If you are looking for an oat-free version, try my Mighty Chia Power Pudding Parfait (see page 225).

   To boost the protein, stir in some good-tasting protein powder, if desired.

Vegan Overnight Oats are the time-crunched person's breakfast secret weapon, since they take just a couple of minutes to make at night before bed. I make Vegan Overnight Oats all the time; nothing is better to wake up to! When you mix together rolled oats, chia seeds and almond milk, the chia seeds absorb the milk and the oats soften, creating an effortless chilled porridge. Place it in the fridge at night and forget about it until morning, when you'll wake up to a cool, creamy bowl of oats that's just perfect in the spring or summer. This is my go-to recipe, but feel free to change up the fruit and other mix-ins as you like.

Serves 3

PREP TIME: 5 minutes • CHILL TIME: overnight

gluten-free, oil-free, raw/no-bake, sugar-free, soy-free

1. In a small bowl, whisk together the oats, almond milk, chia seeds, banana and cinnamon. Cover and refrigerate overnight to thicken.

2. In the morning, stir the oat mixture to combine. Serve the oats in a jar or parfait dish, alternating with layers of fresh fruit (such as mixed berries), granola, hemp seeds and a drizzle of sweetener, if desired.

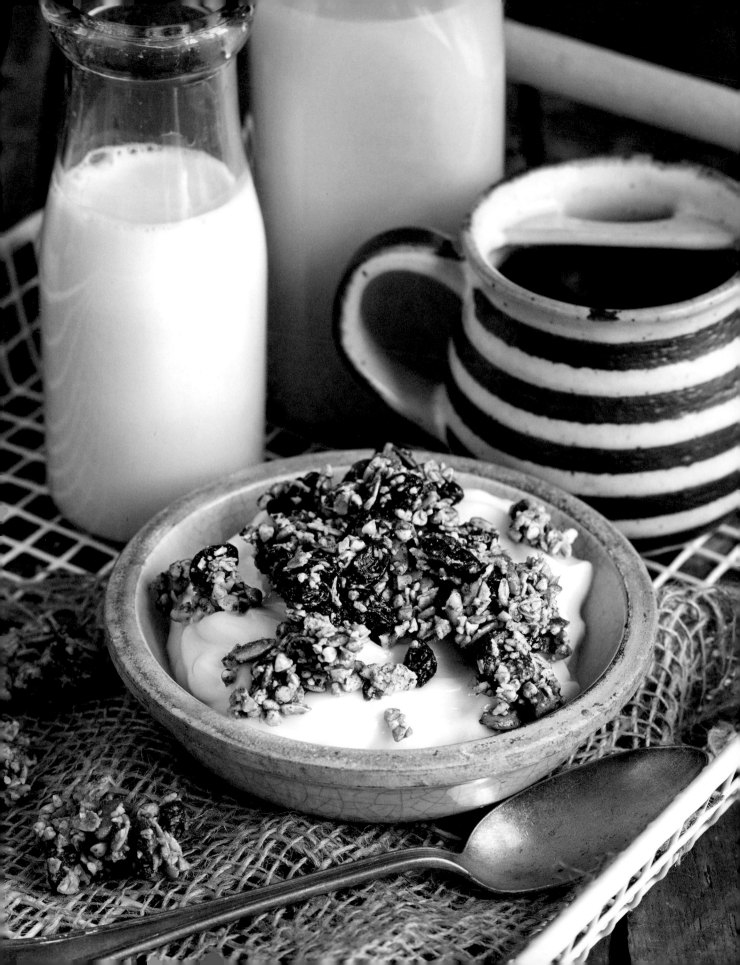

ultimate nutty granola clusters

140g whole raw almonds

50g raw walnut halves or pieces

75g gluten-free rolled oats

50g raw buckwheat groats or gluten-free rolled oats

100g mixed dried fruit (such as cranberries, apricots, cherries, etc.)

65g raw pepita seeds

35g raw sunflower seeds

30g shredded unsweetened coconut

2 teaspoons ground cinnamon

¼ teaspoon fine-grain sea salt

90ml plus 2 tablespoons pure maple syrup or other liquid sweetener

60ml coconut oil, melted

2 teaspoons pure vanilla extract

I drove myself a bit crazy testing this granola recipe. You see, I wanted to create something truly unique, something unlike the loose granola recipes that I had tried. My goal was to create the ultimate nutty, cluster-filled granola. My husband and I ate our weight in granola for weeks on end, but I finally created the perfect granola. It was a tough job, but someone had to do it! Two tips for creating the clusters: Use almond meal to aid binding, and let the granola cool completely on the pan before you break it apart. I know it's a lot to ask, but letting it cool allows the sugars to harden, making it less likely that you'll be left with a crumbly mess at the end. Go ahead and break some off when it comes out of the oven, but leave the rest on the pan for about one hour, and you'll be rewarded with the perfect bite-size clusters for sprinkling on oatmeal, cereal, parfaits and smoothies, or enjoying alone as a snack. This is a versatile recipe, so have fun changing up the nuts, seeds, dried fruit and sweeteners at your every whim.

Makes eighteen 75ml servings

PREP TIME: 15 minutes   •   COOK TIME: 38 to 45 minutes

gluten-free, refined sugar-free, soy-free, grain-free option

1. Preheat the oven to 140°C (275°F). Line a large rimmed baking sheet with parchment paper.

2. Place 70g of the almonds into a food processor and process for about 10 seconds, until a fine meal forms (similar in texture to sand). Transfer the almond meal to a large bowl.

3. In the food processor, combine the remaining almonds and all of the walnuts and process for about 5 seconds, until finely chopped. You'll be left with some larger pieces and some powdery meal,

which is what you want. Add the mixture to the bowl with the almond meal.

4. Add the oats, buckwheat groats, dried fruit, pepita seeds, sunflower seeds, coconut, cinnamon and salt to the large mixing bowl and stir to combine.

5. Add the maple syrup, melted oil, and vanilla to the bowl with the dry ingredients and stir until thoroughly combined.

6. With a spatula, spread the granola into a 1cm layer on the prepared baking sheet and gently press down to compact it slightly. Bake for 20 minutes, then rotate the pan and bake for 18 to 25 minutes more, or until the granola is lightly golden on the bottom and firm to the touch.

7. Cool the granola on the pan for at least 1 hour before breaking it apart into clusters.

8. Store the granola in a glass jar in the fridge for 2 to 3 weeks or freeze it for 4 to 5 weeks.

Tip: If you'd like to make a completely grain-free granola, simply replace the buckwheat groats and rolled oats with an additional 100g finely chopped nuts.

sunrise scramble with
roasted home fries & avocado toast

FOR THE ROASTED HOME FRIES:

1 large russet potato, unpeeled

1 medium sweet potato, unpeeled

1 tablespoon arrowroot powder or cornstarch

¼ teaspoon fine-grain sea salt

1½ teaspoons coconut oil, melted, or grapeseed oil

FOR THE TOFU SCRAMBLE:

2 teaspoons extra-virgin olive oil

2 cloves garlic, minced

2 shallots, thinly sliced, or 75g diced onions

100g sliced cremini mushrooms

1 red bell pepper, seeded and finely chopped

130g destemmed kale leaves or baby spinach, finely chopped

1 tablespoon nutritional yeast (optional)

¼ teaspoon smoked paprika

1 450g package firm or extra-firm tofu, pressed (see page 285)

½ teaspoon fine-grain sea salt

Freshly ground black pepper

¼ teaspoon red pepper flakes (optional)

FOR THE AVOCADO TOAST:

Mashed avocado

Toasted sliced bread (use gluten-free if necessary)

Flaxseed oil or extra-virgin olive oil

Fine-grain sea salt and freshly ground black pepper

Red pepper flakes (optional)

This is a lovely, lazy weekend breakfast featuring scrambled tofu. If you've never had scrambled tofu before, I can promise you it tastes much better than it sounds! When tofu is crumbled and seasoned with spices like smoked paprika and nutritional yeast, it makes a fantastic high-protein replacement for scrambled eggs. Even my husband, Eric, was surprised by how much he enjoyed this breakfast. We like to serve it with roasted potatoes and avocado toast for a filling, stick-to-your-ribs weekend meal.

Serves 4

PREP TIME: 25 minutes • COOK TIME: 30 to 40 minutes

gluten-free, nut-free, sugar-free, grain-free option

1. Make the Roasted Home Fries: Preheat the oven to 220°C (425°F). Line a large rimmed baking sheet with parchment paper.

2. Dice the russet and sweet potatoes into 1cm or smaller pieces. The smaller you chop the potatoes, the faster they will cook.

3. In a large bowl, combine the diced potatoes, the arrowroot powder and the salt and stir to combine. Stir in the coconut oil and mix until thoroughly combined.

4. Spread the potatoes into an even layer on the prepared baking sheet. Bake for 15 minutes, then flip the potatoes and bake for 15 to 25 minutes more, or until crispy, golden brown, and fork-tender.

5. Make the Tofu Scramble: In a large wok, combine the oil, garlic, shallots, and mushrooms and sauté over a medium-high heat for 5 to 10 minutes, until most of the liquid released by the mushrooms has evaporated. Add the bell pepper, kale, nutritional yeast (if using), and smoked paprika. Stir well and continue cooking over a medium-high heat.

6. Crumble or finely chop the tofu and add it to the wok. Stir well to combine. Reduce the heat to medium and sauté for about 10 minutes more. Season with salt, black pepper, and red pepper flakes, if desired. If the mixture becomes dry at any point, you can add a splash of vegetable broth to moisten it, and reduce the heat as needed.

7. Make the Avocado Toast: Spread the mashed avocado on the toast. Top with a drizzle of flaxseed oil and a sprinkle of salt, black pepper, and red pepper flakes, if desired.

8. Plate and serve the home fries, tofu scramble, and toast. Serve with a Flu-Fighter Sunshine Smoothie (page 65), Morning Glory Smoothie (page 66), or orange juice, if desired.

Tips: Leftover tofu scramble is great stuffed into a pita for a quick lunch. Add some salsa and avocado, and you are good to go!

For a grain-free option, omit the avocado toast. For a fun way to change up home fries, try parsnips instead of potatoes.

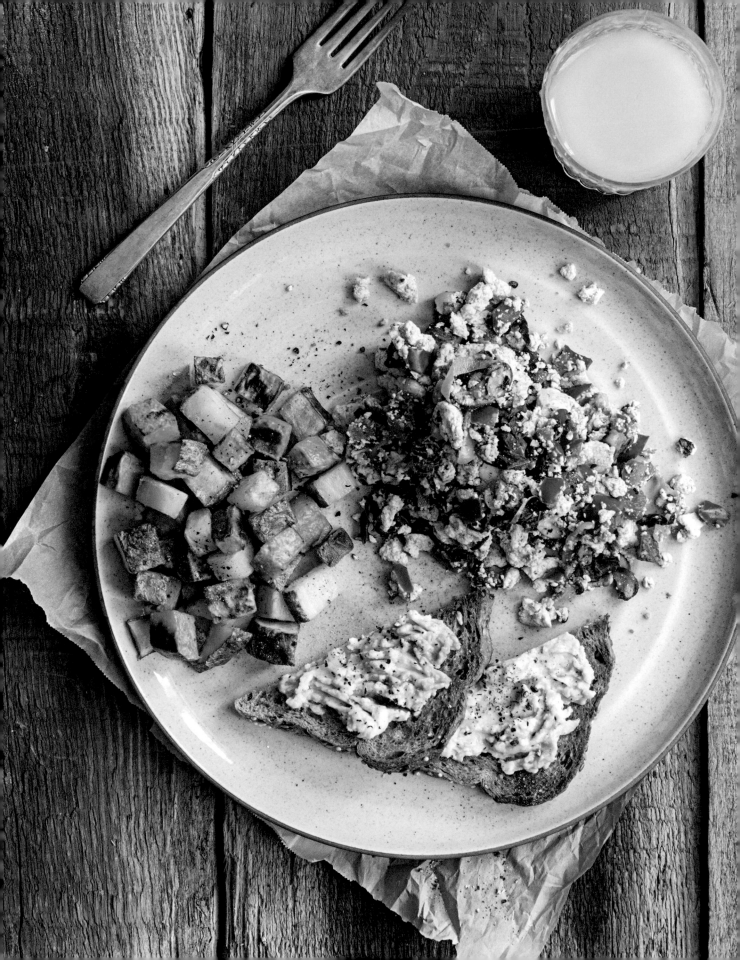

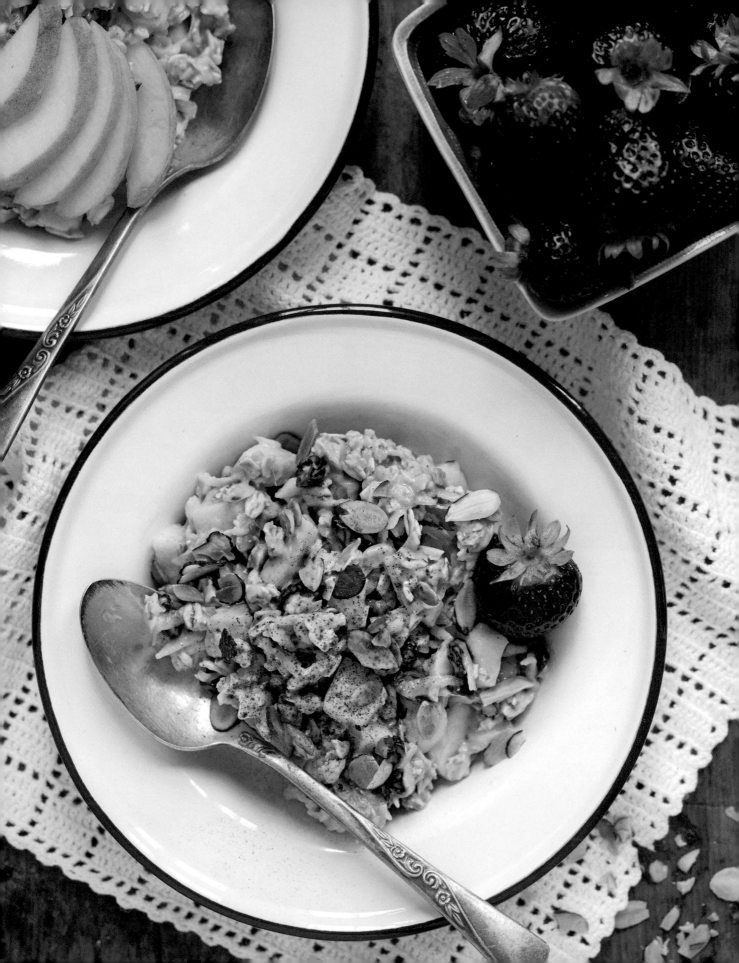

spa day bircher muesli

2 medium apples, peeled and cored

100g gluten-free rolled oats

250ml almond or coconut yoghurt

2 tablespoons raw pepita seeds

2 tablespoons raisins

2 tablespoons dried cranberries

FOR SERVING:
Fresh seasonal fruit

Sliced almonds or other nuts, toasted, if preferred

Pure maple syrup

Cinnamon

Do you ever want to take a spa day in the comfort of your own home? Well, now it's possible with this Spa Day Bircher Muesli! This healthy and filling breakfast takes just a few minutes of preparation before you head to bed. While you get your beauty sleep, the muesli soaks in the fridge, allowing the yoghurt to soften the oats and the flavours to meld. The result is a lightly sweet, super-creamy bowl of chilled oats. In the morning, all you have to do is add a few toppings and then kick back and pamper your health with this delightful breakfast. Feel free to change up the mix-ins to your heart's content; nuts like walnuts would be a nice substitute for the almonds, as would seeds like sunflower, sesame, chia, or flaxseed. Seasonal fruit is a must in my mind. It adds just the right amount of natural sweetness to this dish.

Serves 2 to 3

PREP TIME: 10 minutes

CHILL TIME: overnight, or for at least 2 hours

gluten-free, oil-free, raw/no-bake, soy-free

1. Dice one apple and grate the other on a box grater. Place the apples in a large bowl and add the oats, yoghurt, pepita seeds, raisins, and cranberries. Stir to combine.

2. Cover the bowl and refrigerate the muesli overnight or for at least 2 hours, until the oats soften.

3. Serve the muesli in a bowl, topped with fresh fruit, nuts, maple syrup, and a pinch of cinnamon.

4. Leftover muesli will keep in an airtight container in the refrigerator for 3 to 4 days.

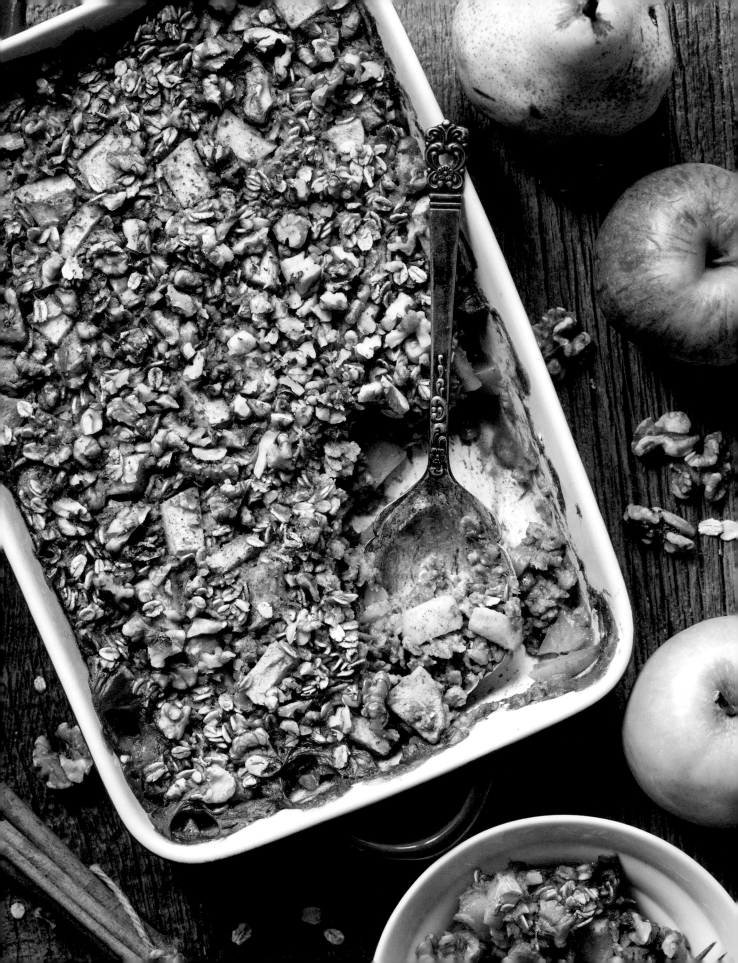

maple-cinnamon
apple & pear baked oatmeal

225g gluten-free rolled oats

2 tablespoons coconut, Sucanat, or brown sugar

2 teaspoons ground cinnamon

1 teaspoon baking powder

½ teaspoon ground ginger

½ teaspoon fine-grain sea salt

½ teaspoon freshly grated nutmeg, or ¼ teaspoon ground nutmeg

500ml unsweetened almond milk

125ml unsweetened apple sauce

65ml pure maple syrup

2 teaspoons pure vanilla extract

2 apples, peeled and diced

1 ripe pear, peeled and diced

50g walnuts, chopped (optional)

Baked oatmeal is one of my favourite lazy weekend breakfasts. This fall-inspired combo of apple, spices, and pear will warm you up on any chilly morning. Try using a tart apple like Granny Smith along with a sweet variety like Gala; the contrast is really nice. I love serving this dish as part of a holiday brunch; it's always a hit. To save time, refrigerate the mixture overnight in a casserole dish so it's ready to throw into the oven when you wake up (see Tip, page 40). It also makes a healthy midday snack or dessert served with a dollop of Whipped Coconut Cream (see page 280). If you'd like to change it up, try replacing the apples with two large ripe bananas and the pear with 150g blueberries.

Serves 6

PREP TIME: 25 to 30 minutes • COOK TIME: 35 to 45 minutes
gluten-free, oil-free, refined sugar-free, soy-free

1. Preheat the oven to 190°C (375°F). Lightly grease a 2 to 2.5-litre casserole dish.

2. In a large bowl, combine the rolled oats, sugar, cinnamon, baking powder, ginger, salt, and nutmeg. Mix well.

3. In a separate bowl, combine the almond milk, apple sauce, maple syrup, and vanilla and stir well to combine.

4. Pour the liquid mixture over the oat mixture and stir until combined. The mixture will have a soupy consistency. Fold in the chopped apples and pear.

5. Spoon the oatmeal mixture into the prepared casserole dish and smooth out the top. Sprinkle the walnuts (if using) on top and gently press them down into the oatmeal with your hands.

6. Bake, uncovered, for 35 to 45 minutes, or until the oatmeal is bubbly around the corners and the apples are fork-tender.

7. Cool the oatmeal for 5 to 10 minutes before serving. Enjoy with a splash of almond milk and a drizzle of maple syrup, if desired.

8. Cool the oatmeal completely before wrapping it up and placing it in an airtight container. It will keep in the fridge for 5 to 6 days or in the freezer for 2 to 3 weeks.

Tips: Enjoy this breakfast warmed or chilled; it's lovely warmed on a chilly morning, but it's also nice straight from the fridge.

To save time in the morning, prepare this oatmeal the night before. Cover the dish and refrigerate the unbaked oatmeal overnight. In the morning, simply preheat the oven and let the oatmeal sit on the counter while the oven gets hot. Uncover and stir the oatmeal mixture gently to redistribute the milk. Smooth out the top, if necessary, and bake as directed.

out-the-door chia
power doughnuts

75g gluten-free oat flour

30g chia seeds

1½ teaspoons baking powder

¼ teaspoon fine-grain sea salt

¼ teaspoon ground cinnamon

75ml pure maple syrup or other liquid sweetener

75ml non-dairy milk

1 teaspoon pure vanilla extract

Coconut-Lemon Whipped Cream (see page 281), for serving

This recipe is proof that not all doughnuts have to be the unhealthy kind. Packed with antioxidants, omega-3 fatty acids, protein, and fibre, these baked doughnuts will have you feeling ready to conquer your day (or the world?). Unlike light and fluffy fried doughnuts, these baked doughnuts are dense, filling, and a bit crunchy, thanks to the generous amount of chia seeds. I've added a decadent, but healthy, Coconut-Lemon Whipped Cream, but it's totally optional. The doughnuts are just as tasty served plain or spread with jam and nut butter. You be the judge.

Makes 6 doughnuts
PREP TIME: 10 minutes
COOK TIME: 22 to 26 minutes
gluten-free, nut-free, oil-free, soy-free, refined sugar free

1. Preheat the oven to 150°C (300°F). Lightly grease a 6-cavity doughnut pan with oil. Set aside.

2. In a large bowl, combine the oat flour, chia seeds, baking powder, salt, and cinnamon.

3. Add the maple syrup, milk, and vanilla and stir until combined. The batter will be very runny, but this is normal.

4. Spoon the batter into the prepared doughnut pan, filling each cavity to the top.

5. Bake the doughnuts for 22 to 26 minutes, until firm to the touch. A toothpick inserted into a doughnut should come out clean.

6. Cool the doughnuts in the pan for about 10 minutes, and then carefully invert the pan onto a cooling rack. The doughnuts should pop right out – if they don't, let them cool a bit more and gently run

a butter knife along the edges of the wells to loosen them. Cool the doughnuts completely on the rack.

7. Drizzle Coconut-Lemon Whipped Cream over top and enjoy. You can also use the whipped cream as a dip if you prefer a travel-friendly option.

Tip: If you don't have a doughnut pan, fear not – a muffin tin will work just fine!

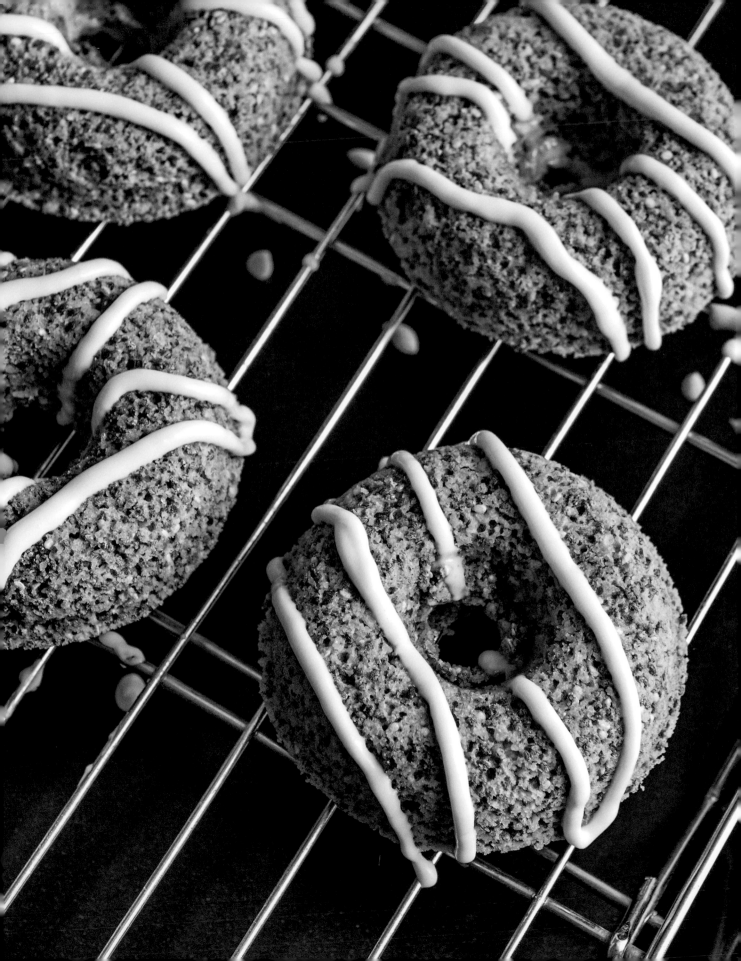

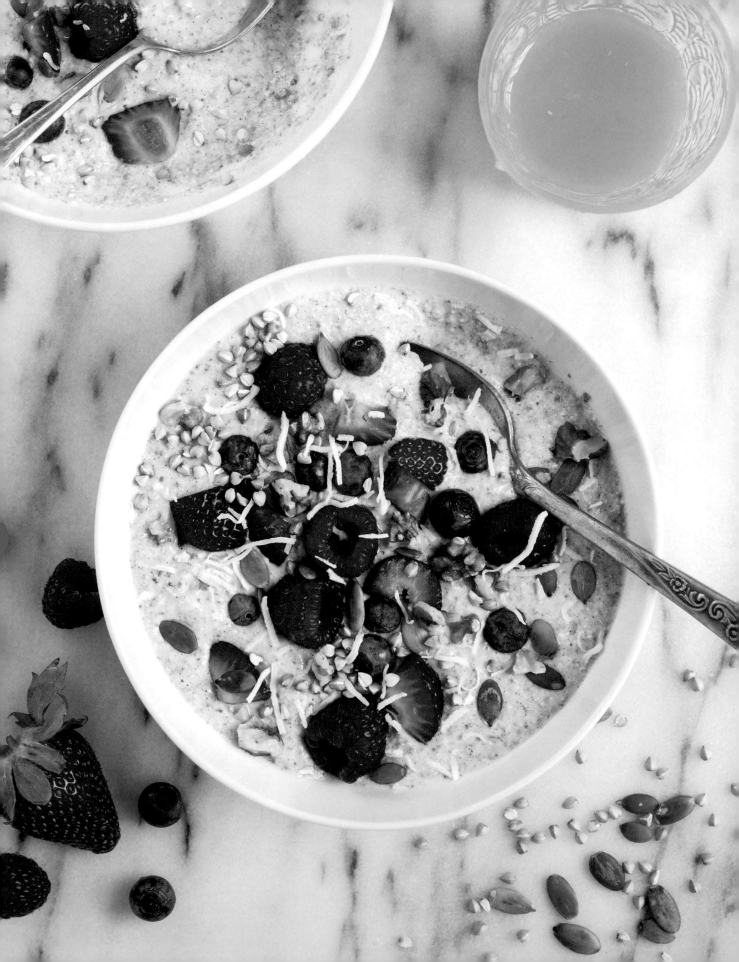

raw buckwheat breakfast porridge

100g raw buckwheat groats

125ml almond milk

1 tablespoon chia seeds

½ teaspoon pure vanilla extract

2 tablespoons liquid sweetener

½ teaspoon ground cinnamon

OPTIONAL TOPPINGS:
Fresh or dried fruit

Chopped nuts and/or seeds

Magical Chia Seed Jam (see page 287)

Nut or seed butter

Toasted unsweetened shredded coconut

Ultimate Nutty Granola Clusters (see page 31)

Chia seeds or ground flaxseed

This is easily one of my all-time favourite breakfast recipes (okay, I have a lot!), and it's one of the most popular breakfast recipes on my blog. When raw buckwheat groats are soaked, they are not only easier to digest but soften up and blend easily with almond milk, a bit of sweetener, vanilla, and cinnamon to create a delicious raw porridge. If you need breakfast on the go, simply place some porridge in a jar, add your desired toppings, screw on the lid, and throw it into your bag with a spoon. Or better yet, prepare and pack it before bed so you can just grab a jar in the morning as you head out the door. Now there's simply no excuse to skip breakfast!

Serves 2

PREP TIME: 10 minutes • SOAK TIME: 1 hour or overnight
gluten-free, oil-free, raw/no-bake, soy-free, refined sugar-free

1. Place the buckwheat groats in a small bowl and add water to cover. Soak the groats overnight or for at least 1 hour at room temperature. The groats will feel a bit slimy after soaking, but this is normal. Drain the groats in a strainer and rinse them thoroughly for at least 1 minute. This will help remove the gelatinous coating that forms on the buckwheat as it soaks.

2. Place the groats in a blender (or food processor) and add the almond milk, chia seeds, and vanilla. Blend the mixture until combined and almost smooth. Add the sweetener and cinnamon and blend briefly just to combine.

3. Scoop the porridge into bowls or parfait glasses and add your desired toppings.

4. Place any leftovers in a sealed container or jar. The porridge will keep in the refrigerator for 3 to 4 days.

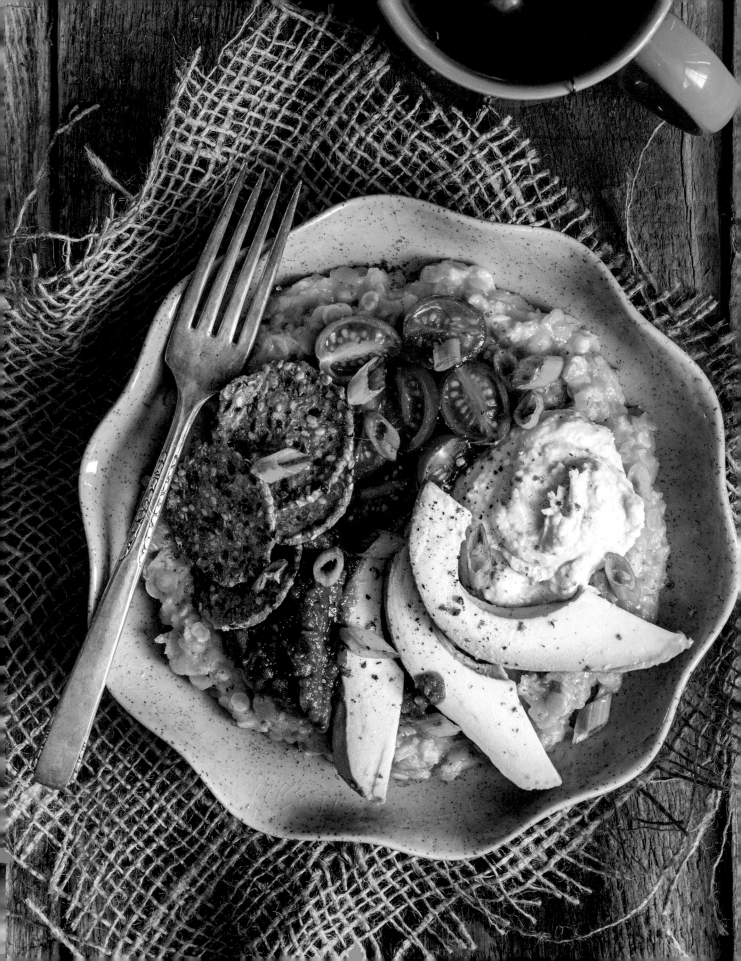

loaded savoury oatmeal & lentil bowl

30g gluten-free rolled oats

30g red lentils

365 to 425ml vegetable broth

1 small clove garlic, minced (optional)

1 small shallot, chopped, or 2 to 3 table-spoons chopped onion (optional)

Fine-grain sea salt and freshly ground black pepper, to taste

OPTIONAL TOPPINGS:
Sliced avocado

Salsa

Chopped green onion

Classic Hummus (see page 89), or store-bought

Crackers

Tip: For a grain-free option, replace the oats with an extra 70g red lentils.

If the thought of something sweet in the morning turns your tummy, this recipe might be right up your alley. If you've never had savoury oatmeal before, I urge you to give this a try. To boost the protein in this recipe, I cooked red lentils with the rolled oats. Red lentils have an ultra-quick cooking time, so they make an effortless add-in to regular oatmeal, and the protein will fill you up and power your morning like nothing else. You can top oats with any savoury ingredients that you love, but I especially enjoy them topped with hummus, salsa, crackers, and avocado. It's fun to build different power bowls depending on your mood! If you can't wrap your head around a savoury dish like this in the morning, feel free to enjoy this recipe as a quick-and-easy cool-weather lunch.

Serves 2

PREP TIME: 10 to 15 minutes • COOK TIME: 8 to 12 minutes
gluten-free, nut-free, oil-free, soy-free, sugar-free, grain-free option

1. In a medium saucepan, combine the oats, lentils, broth, garlic (if using), and shallot (if using). Bring the mixture to a low boil over a medium-high heat, then reduce the heat to medium-low and simmer, uncovered, for 8 to 12 minutes, or until thickened. Season with salt and pepper to taste.

2. Spoon the oatmeal into a bowl, add your desired toppings, and enjoy!

3. Store any leftovers in an airtight container. They will keep in the refrigerator for 2 to 3 days. To reheat, simply combine the oatmeal and a splash of vegetable broth in a small saucepan and heat over medium-low heat until warmed through.

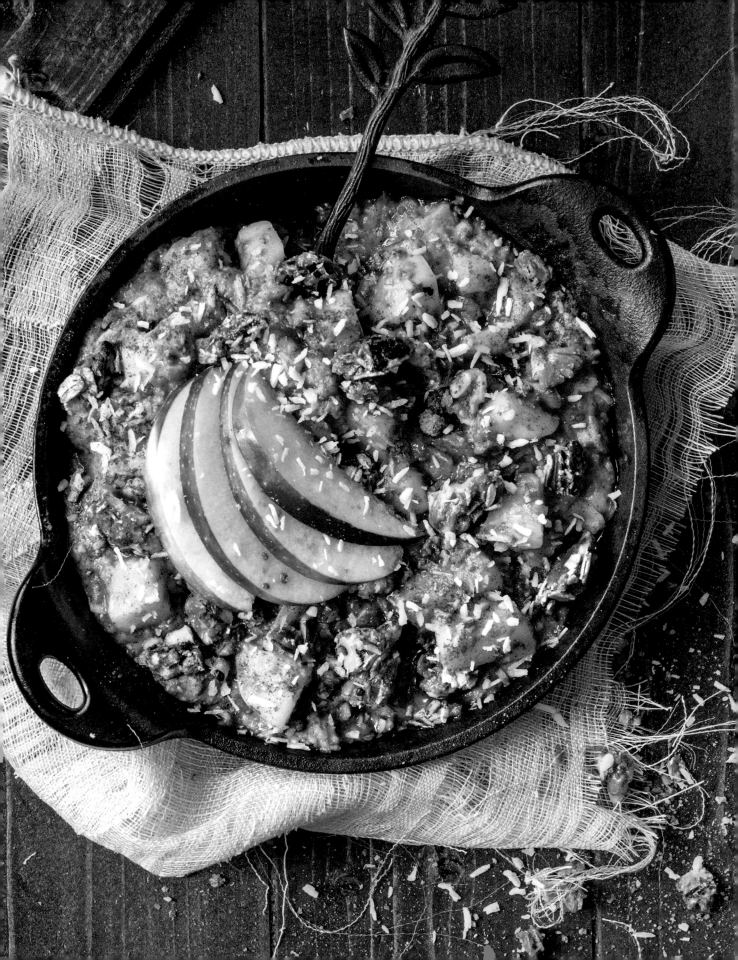

apple pie oatmeal

30g gluten-free rolled oats

1 medium Gala apple, peeled, cored, and chopped into 2.5cm pieces

1 tablespoon chia seeds

125ml unsweetened apple sauce

250ml almond milk

1 teaspoon ground cinnamon, plus more for serving

¼ teaspoon ground ginger

Pinch of fine-grain sea salt

½ teaspoon pure vanilla extract

1 tablespoon pure maple syrup, to taste, plus more for serving

1 tablespoon chopped walnuts, for serving

1 tablespoon hemp seeds, for serving

Pinch of unsweetened shredded coconut, for serving

This voluminous Apple Pie Oatmeal will remind you of delicious apple pie, but will leave you feeling energized and ready to tackle the day ahead. I like Gala apples in this recipe, but feel free to use any variety that you wish.

Serves 1

PREP TIME: 15 minutes • COOK TIME: 8 to 12 minutes

gluten-free, oil-free, refined sugar-free, soy-free

1. In a medium saucepan, over a medium heat, combine the oats, apple, chia seeds, apple sauce, almond milk, cinnamon, ginger, and salt. Whisk well to combine. Bring the mixture to a low boil over medium heat. Simmer for 8 to 10 minutes, stirring often.

2. When the mixture has thickened and the liquid has been absorbed, remove the pan from the heat and stir in the vanilla and maple syrup to taste.

3. Pour the oatmeal into a bowl and top it with chopped walnuts, hemp seeds, a pinch of cinnamon, a pinch of shredded coconut, and a drizzle of pure maple syrup.

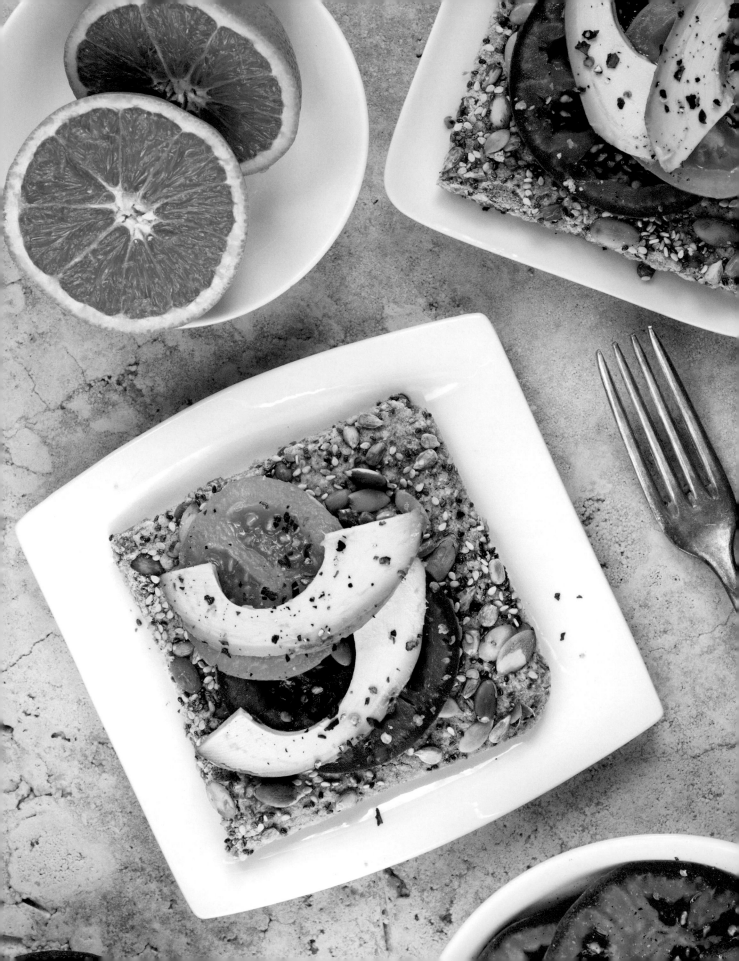

crunchy seed & oat flatbread

FOR THE SEED TOPPING:

4 teaspoons raw pepita seeds

1 tablespoon raw sunflower seeds

½ teaspoon chia seeds

½ teaspoon sesame seeds

Herbamare or fine-grain sea salt, for sprinkling

FOR THE FLATBREAD:

75g gluten-free rolled oats

50g raw buckwheat groats

35g raw sunflower seeds

1 tablespoon chia seeds

1½ teaspoons granulated sugar

1 teaspoon dried oregano

¼ teaspoon dried thyme

¼ teaspoon baking powder

¼ teaspoon garlic powder

¼ teaspoon fine-grain sea salt

250ml unsweetened and unflavoured non-dairy milk

1 tablespoon coconut oil, melted, or olive oil

Not only is this flatbread gluten- and yeast-free, but you can throw it together in just a few minutes. A far cry from light and fluffy bread, this flatbread is dense, filling, and sturdy enough to pop into the toaster. The seeds give it a fantastic crunch, adding healthy fats and a great chewy texture. One large piece has 8 grams of protein and 6 grams of fibre, making it a bread that will power you through your day! Try toasting a slice and topping it with avocado, hummus, and tomato for a tasty open-faced sandwich, or enjoy it with nut butter and jam to start your day.

Serves 4

PREP TIME: 10 minutes • BAKE TIME: 25 to 30 minutes

gluten-free, nut-free, soy-free

1. Preheat the oven to 180°C (350°F). Lightly grease a 2.5-litre square pan and line it with two pieces of parchment paper, one going each way.

2. Make the Seed Topping: In a small bowl, combine the pepita, sunflower, chia, and sesame seeds and stir to combine. Set aside.

3. Make the Flatbread: In a high-speed blender, combine the oats and buckwheat and blend on high until a flour forms, 5 to 10 seconds.

4. In a large bowl, combine the oat and buckwheat flour, sunflower seeds, chia seeds, sugar, oregano, thyme, baking powder, garlic powder, and salt. Whisk to combine.

5. Add the milk and oil to the bowl and stir very well until no clumps remain. Immediately pour the batter into the prepared pan and smooth it out with a spatula.

6. Sprinkle the batter evenly with the prepared seed topping and the Herbamare. Lightly press down on the topping with your hands to adhere it to the batter.

7. Bake for 25 to 30 minutes, uncovered, until the flatbread is firm to the touch.

8. Let the flatbread cool in the pan placed on a cooling rack for 15 minutes. Lift it out of the pan and place it on a clean work surface. Using a pizza cutter, slice it into 4 squares (or any number you wish).

9. Store the flatbread in an airtight container in the refrigerator for up to 2 days. It can be frozen for up to 2 weeks.

Tip: This bread is fantastic toasted. Gently shake off any loose seeds before toasting to prevent them from falling into the toaster and burning. I love topping a toasted slice with sunflower seed butter and jam!

smoothies, juice & tea

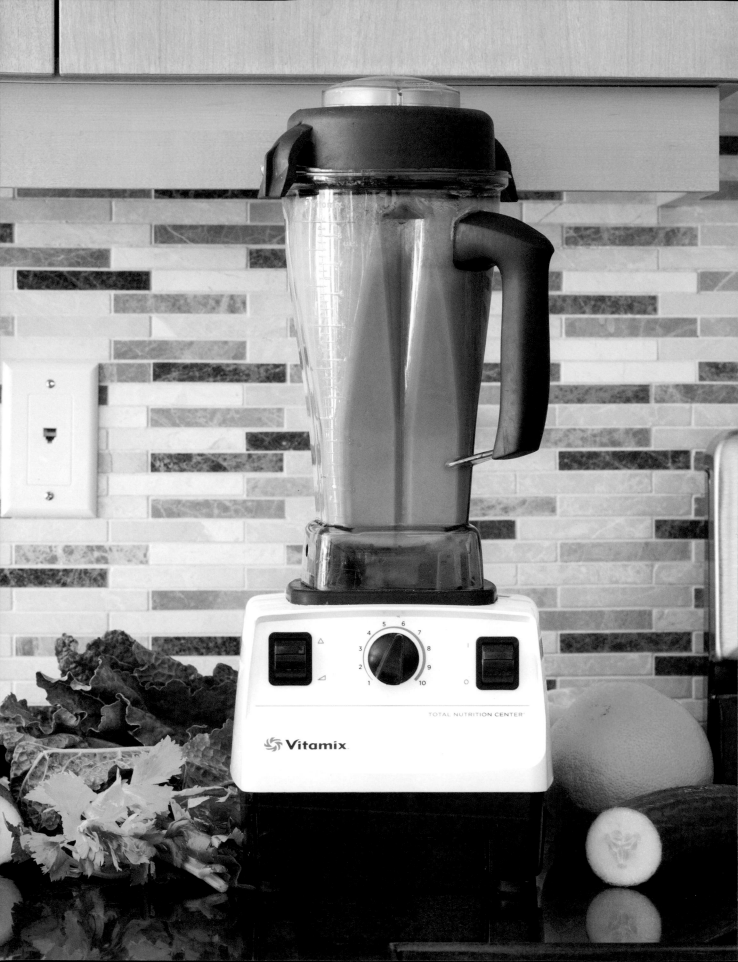

I first started experimenting with smoothies in 2009 after Eric and I received a blender as a wedding gift. At the time, I wasn't a big smoothie fan so it took me a few months to even crack open the box, but once I did, I soon got hooked. Little did I know that a blender would set the tone for a huge change in my diet! I started tossing all kinds of greens, fruit, and other veggies into my blender, and I drank whatever crazy mixture came out. Some combinations were great, some weren't. Luckily, my smoothie-making skills improved over time and I also came to appreciate how easy it was to enjoy several servings of fruit and veggies all in one drink. I still believe there is no better (or quicker) way to get a huge dose of nutrients in one serving.

It helps to do a bit of smoothie prep in advance to streamline your smoothie making. Once a week, I peel, chop, and freeze several bananas so I have frozen bananas ready to go. You can also prep and freeze other fruits, like mango, berries, or pineapple, so you always have frozen fruit on hand, or simply buy frozen fruit to save time. Another time-saving step is to rinse large batches of greens (such as kale and spinach) and then freeze them so they stay fresh and are ready when you need them.

I love having a smoothie every single day and can't imagine my life without them. Whether you are a fellow smoothie addict, tea drinker, or juice lover, there is something for everyone in this chapter, from my Cheerful Chocolate Smoothie (page 61) to my Metabolism-Boosting Green Citrus Tea (page 73). Cheers to glowing good health!

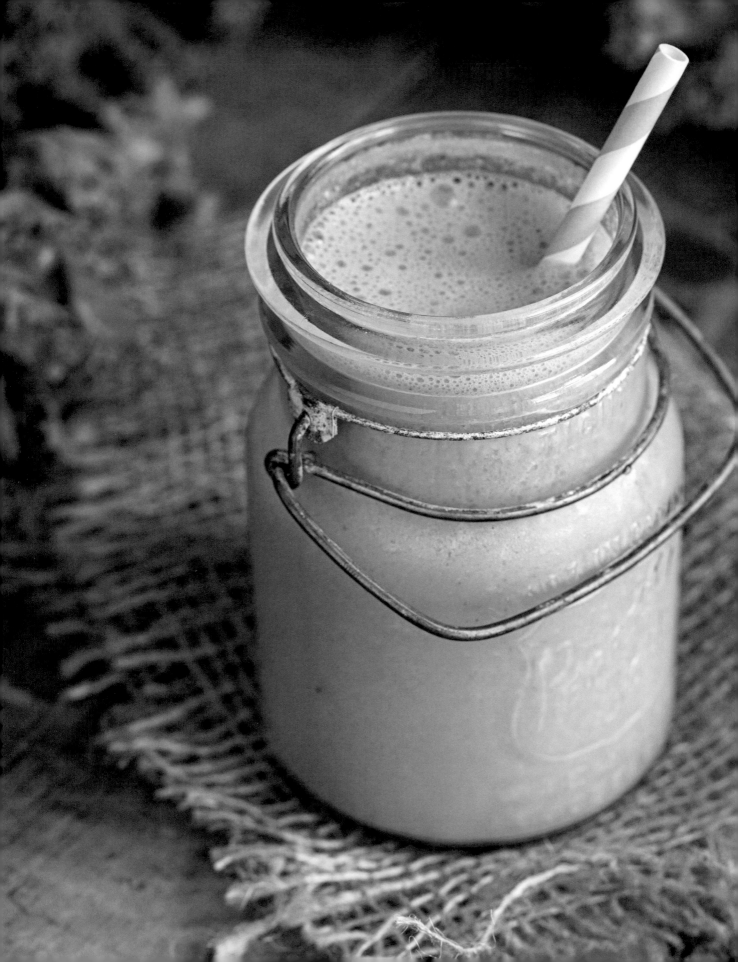

classic green monster

250ml almond milk or other
non-dairy milk

65g destemmed kale leaves or baby
spinach

1 ripe banana, peeled and frozen

2 to 3 ice cubes

1 tablespoon almond butter or peanut
butter

1 tablespoon pure chia seeds or ground
flaxseed

¼ teaspoon pure vanilla extract

Pinch of ground cinnamon

Protein powder (optional)

Tips: It's easy to make a double batch
and refrigerate the leftovers in a jar for
the next day. Or, prepare the smoothie
at night and store it in the fridge for
the next morning. Sometimes I do this
if time is tight in the morning or if I
have sleeping houseguests around. No
one likes to be woken up by a Vitamix,
my cat included.

   To make this nut-free, use coconut
milk and sunflower seed butter instead
of almond milk and nut butter.

Adding greens to smoothies is a trend you see everywhere these
days, but when I first started adding spinach to my smoothies in
2009, many of my blog readers, family members, and coworkers
were both horrified and intrigued by the weird-looking drinks that
gave me so much energy. Of course, my first attempts were a bit
scary-looking, which is why I called them 'Green Monsters', but
eventually I started blending up delicious concoctions, sharing the
recipes on my blog, and gushing about how much I loved them. I
never once expected Green Monsters to become such a sensation,
but soon readers from all over the world sent in recipes and pictures
of their own green smoothies. To this day, Green Monsters are one
of my favourite drinks for glowing skin and increased energy. If you
are a newbie, feel free to start off with baby spinach since its taste is
undetectable, but I encourage you to experiment with kale, romaine
lettuce, or other leafy greens as well. It's common to find many
'power green' blends in the produce aisle, which are great options,
too. Just be sure to use a sturdy high-speed blender that can handle
the task of blending thick greens.

   For those of you who aren't fans of drinking something green,
simply add 50g frozen or fresh blueberries to this smoothie to give it
a beautiful purple hue.

Makes 1 375 to 500ml smoothie
PREP TIME: 5 minutes
*gluten-free, oil-free, raw/no-bake, sugar-free, soy-free,
grain-free, nut-free option*

1. In a high-speed blender, combine all of the ingredients and blend
until smooth.

2. Serve immediately and enjoy a burst of energy any time of the
day!

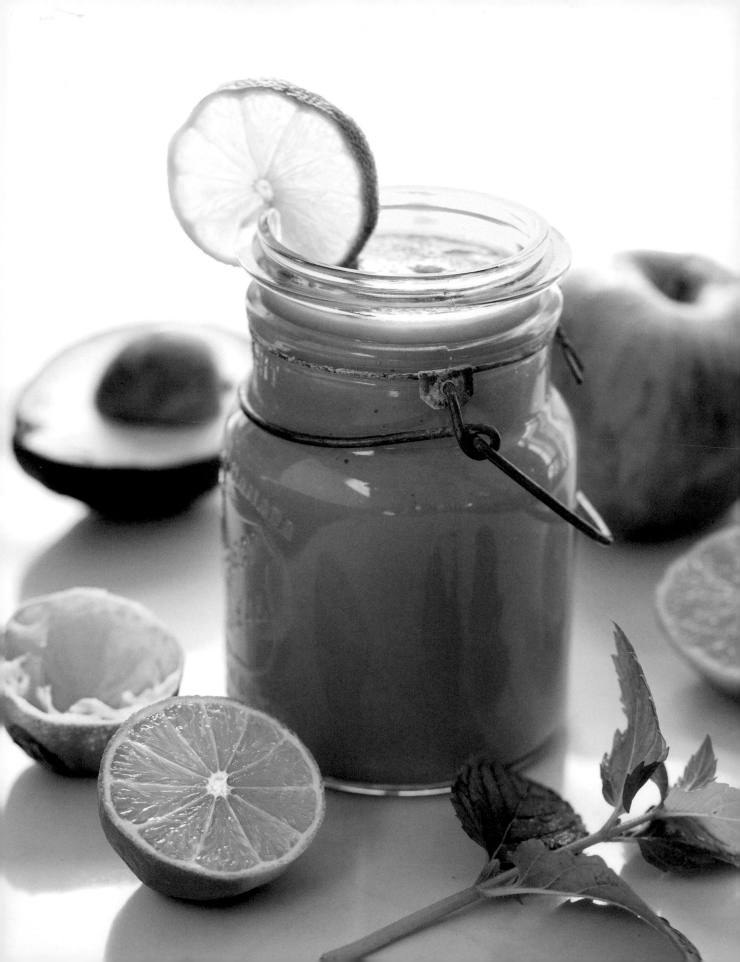

glowing mojo-ito green monster

75g watermelon cubes (optional, but recommended)

30 to 50g baby spinach or other leafy greens

250ml coconut water or water

1 large sweet apple (such as Gala or Honeycrisp)

3 tablespoons avocado

1 to 2 tablespoons fresh lime juice, to taste

5 to 10 large mint leaves, to taste

5 large ice cubes

Like a party in your glass, this energizing mint, creamy avocado, and zesty lime smoothie is the perfect refreshing drink to win over any green smoothie sceptic. Invite your friends over, serve up a double or triple batch of this Green Monster, and toast to glowing energy and health. If you are feeling wild, add a splash of sparkling water (and optional white rum) to make an alternative to a classic mojito.

Makes 1 750ml smoothie

PREP TIME: 5 minutes

gluten-free, oil-free, raw/no-bake, soy-free, sugar-free, grain-free, nut-free

1. Freeze the watermelon cubes (if using) overnight or until frozen solid.

2. In a high-speed blender, combine all of the ingredients and blend until smooth. Pour into a glass and toast to green drinks!

Tip: If using water instead of coconut water, you might want to add a bit of liquid sweetener to make up for the lack of sweetness.

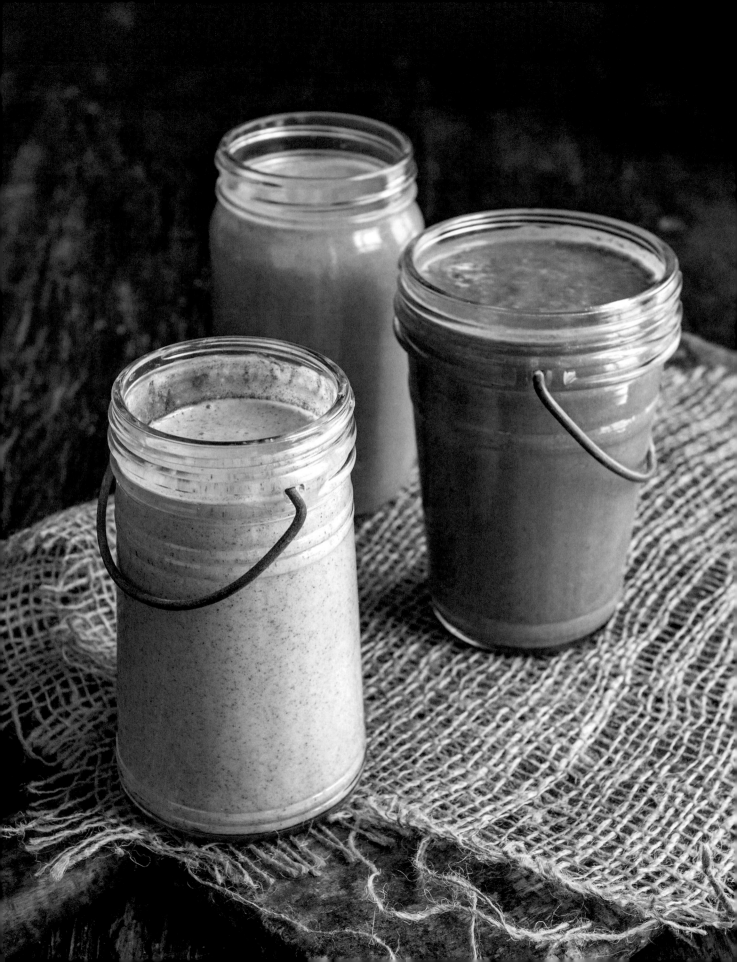

cheerful chocolate smoothie

500ml almond milk

40g avocado

2 tablespoons unsweetened cocoa powder

1 teaspoon pure vanilla extract

Very small pinch of fine-grain sea salt

4 to 6 pitted medium Medjool dates,
to taste

4 to 6 ice cubes

¼ teaspoon espresso powder (optional)

Is there anything more cheerful than chocolate? I think not! And the avocado in this smoothie gives it a luxurious, creamy texture while adding a nice boost of healthy fats. I tested this smoothie multiple times to find the right consistency and flavour, and 40g of avocado was perfection. If avocado isn't your thing, however, feel free to substitute one frozen banana in its place. This light brown smoothie also masks the colour of spinach quite well, so if you'd like to 'hide' some greens, feel free to add a handful! Your kids – or spouse – probably won't be the wiser. (If this were an audiobook, you'd hear me cackling right now.) To change up this smoothie, add 1 tablespoon of peanut butter or almond butter.

Makes 2 500ml smoothies

PREP TIME: 5 minutes

gluten-free, oil-free, raw/no-bake, soy-free,
sugar-free, grain-free, nut-free option

1. In a high-speed blender, combine the almond milk, avocado, cocoa powder, and vanilla and blend on high speed until smooth.

2. Add the salt, pitted dates, ice, and espresso powder (if using). Blend again until smooth.

Tips: Instead of regular ice cubes, try using coffee ice cubes for this smoothie. They add an incredible mocha flavour that would rival a popular drink from a high-end coffee shop!

If you have leftover avocado, you can freeze it for 1 to 2 weeks and use it for future smoothies.

If your dates are firm, be sure to soak them in a bowl of water to soften before use.

For a nut-free version, substitute a nut-free, non-dairy milk (such as coconut) for the almond milk.

FRONT TO BACK:
Gym Rat Smoothie,
Cheerful Chocolate Smoothie,
Velvety Pumpkin Pie Smoothie

velvety pumpkin pie smoothie

250ml almond milk

2 tablespoons gluten-free rolled oats

125g canned pure pumpkin

½ to 1 teaspoon blackstrap molasses, to taste

½ large banana, frozen

1 teaspoon ground cinnamon, plus more for serving (optional)

¼ teaspoon ground ginger

⅛ teaspoon freshly grated nutmeg

4 or 5 ice cubes

1 tablespoon pure maple syrup

Whipped Coconut Cream (see page 280), for serving (optional)

Every October, I go absolutely crazy over pumpkin for approximately two months, and then the rest of the year I don't want anything to do with it. Poor, sweet pumpkin. During my pumpkin craze, I can't get enough of this decadent pumpkin pie smoothie. Packed with 115g pumpkin per serving, this smoothie has a delicious pumpkin pie flavour while giving you a good dose of vitamins A and C and lots of fibre. Fresh-cooked pumpkin and butternut squash also work beautifully in this smoothie, so feel free to use fresh if you have some on hand.

Makes 1 500ml smoothie
PREP TIME: 10 minutes
gluten-free, oil-free, raw/no-bake, soy-free, refined sugar free, grain-free option, nut-free option

1. In a high-speed blender, combine the milk, oats, pumpkin, molasses, banana, cinnamon, ginger, and nutmeg. Blend on high speed until smooth. Add the ice cubes and blend until ice cold.

2. Add the maple syrup and blend briefly to combine.

3. Serve topped with Whipped Coconut Cream and a sprinkle of cinnamon, if desired.

Tips: If your blender has a difficult time blending rolled oats, place the oats and milk in the blender, stir, and let sit for 10 to 15 minutes to soften. Then proceed with your smoothie making. This will help the mixture blend more smoothly.

For a grain-free option, omit rolled oats.

For a nut-free version, swap the almond milk for a nut-free, non-dairy milk like coconut milk.

gym rat smoothie

250ml almond milk

2 tablespoons gluten-free rolled oats

2 to 3 pitted Medjool dates, to taste

1 tablespoon chia seeds

1 tablespoon peanut butter or almond butter

¼ to ½ teaspoon ground cinnamon, to taste

¼ teaspoon pure vanilla extract

4 to 5 ice cubes

When I dream about my favourite splurge-worthy smoothies, I dream about this peanut butter, cinnamon, and date smoothie. Bursting with creamy peanut butter and almond milk, it's naturally sweetened with dates, making this a smoothie you can feel good about guzzling down. Although this drink already boasts more than 8 grams protein, you can easily add a scoop of vanilla protein powder to bring it up to more than 20 grams protein for a great post-workout recovery drink.

Makes 1 425ml smoothie

PREP TIME: 5 minutes

*gluten-free, oil-free, raw/no-bake, soy-free, sugar-free,
grain-free option, nut-free option*

1. In a high-speed blender, combine all of the ingredients and blend until smooth.

Tips: If your blender has a difficult time pureeing rolled oats and dates, place the oats, pitted dates, and almond milk in the blender, stir, and let sit for 10 to 15 minutes to soften. Then proceed with your smoothie making. This will help the mixture blend more smoothly.

For a grain-free option, omit the rolled oats.

For a nut-free version, swap the almond milk for a nut-free, non-dairy milk like coconut milk and the peanut butter for sunflower seed butter.

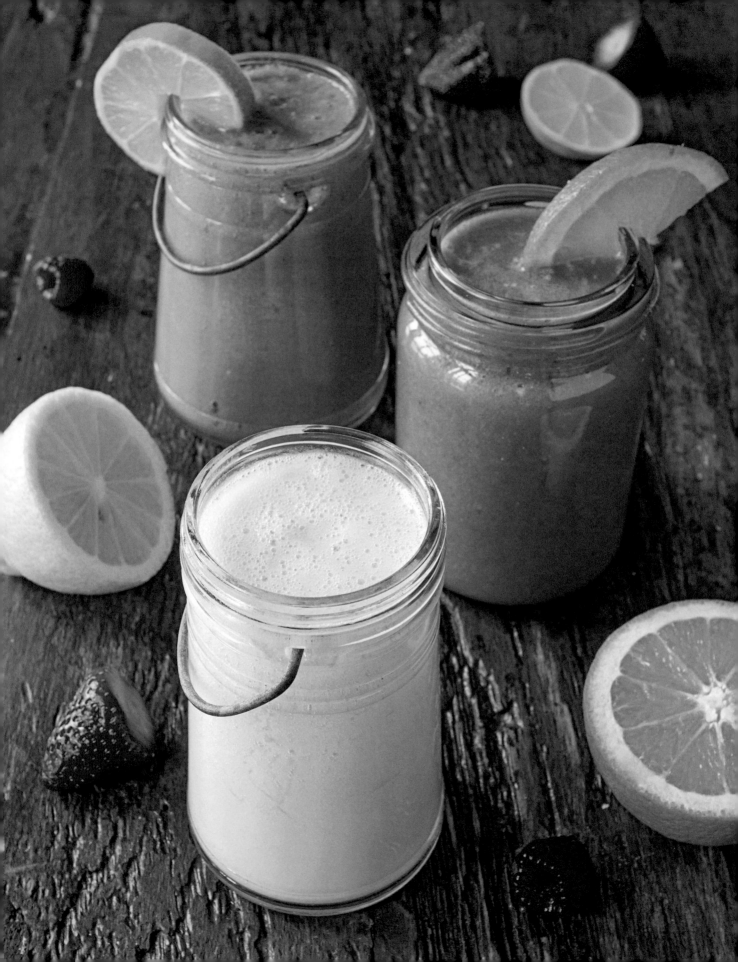

flu-fighter sunshine smoothie

2 medium seedless navel oranges, peeled

2 tablespoons fresh lemon juice, or
to taste

1 teaspoon grated peeled fresh ginger, or
to taste

1 to 3 teaspoons pure maple syrup, to taste

3 to 5 ice cubes

Pinch of cayenne pepper (optional)

I created this vibrant yellow smoothie when I had a nasty flu and was desperate to get better. Antioxidant-packed citrus fruit and fresh ginger unite to kick any cold or flu's behind. If you're feeling really desperate, like I was, add a small amount of cayenne pepper to the mix. You'll be breathing free and clear in no time! Word on the street is that cayenne pepper also boosts your metabolism.

Makes 1 425ml smoothie
PREP TIME: 10 minutes
gluten-free, nut-free, oil-free, raw/no-bake,
soy-free, refined sugar-free, grain-free

1. In a high-speed blender, combine all of the ingredients and blend until smooth. Drink and get ready to feel better in a flash.

Tips: If you'd like this smoothie served warm, omit the ice and keep blending on high speed for a few minutes, until the heat of the blender motor warms the mixture.

For even more nutritional power, try adding a bit of kale or spinach into the mix!

FRONT TO BACK:
Flu-Fighter Sunshine Smoothie,
Morning Glory Smoothie,
Tropical Beauty Green Monster

morning glory smoothie

200g fresh or frozen strawberries, hulled

1 frozen banana, roughly chopped

75ml fresh orange juice

75ml coconut water or water

¼ teaspoon pure vanilla extract (optional)

3 to 5 ice cubes

My husband, Eric, is quite the smoothie connoisseur, or at least he was during the development of this smoothie chapter. I challenged myself to come up with a smoothie he could call his all-time favourite for this book, and I'm embarrassed to tell you how many trials it took to win his approval. I almost threw in the tea towel! Finally, a miracle happened and he fell in love with this manly pink combo of strawberries, banana, orange juice, and vanilla. It's a simple mix, but he's a pretty simple guy! Try serving this smoothie as part of a lazy Sunday morning brunch; the recipe can be easily doubled or tripled depending on how many thirsty guests you are serving.

Makes 1 500ml smoothie

PREP TIME: 5 minutes

gluten-free, nut-free, oil-free, raw/no-bake, soy-free, sugar-free, grain-free

1. In a high-speed blender, combine all of the ingredients and blend until smooth.

tropical beauty green monster

250ml coconut water or water

65g destemmed kale leaves or baby spinach

200g frozen mango, or 1 fresh mango, chopped

100g fresh or frozen pineapple chunks

1 to 2 tablespoons fresh lime juice, to taste

1 teaspoon minced peeled fresh ginger

Liquid sweetener, to taste (optional)

Ice cubes, if desired

If you can't get away for a vacation but still want a taste of the tropics, this smoothie is for you. Filled with coconut water, mango, pineapple, and lime, all you need to do is close your eyes and you'll be transported to a sunny, white-sand beach. Oh, and don't be surprised if you come back with a little 'post-vacation' glow!

Makes 1 500ml smoothie

PREP TIME: 5 minutes

gluten-free, oil-free, raw/no-bake, soy-free,
refined sugar-free, grain-free, nut-free

1. In a high-speed blender, combine all of the ingredients and blend until smooth. Add a drink umbrella to get the party started!

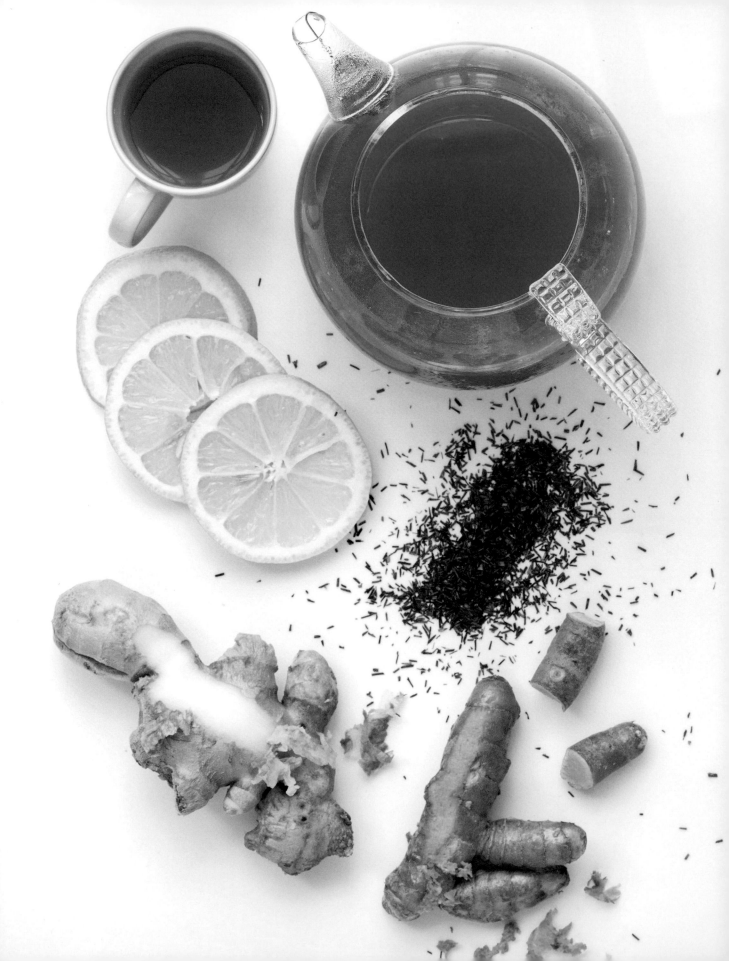

healing rooibos tea

1 litre filtered water

4 teaspoons loose rooibos tea, or 4 rooibos tea bags

1 to 2 lemon slices, seeds removed

2.5 to 5cm piece turmeric root, peeled and thinly sliced

5 to 8cm piece fresh ginger, peeled and thinly sliced

Sweetener, to taste (optional)

Tips: To peel ginger and turmeric easily, use a grapefruit spoon to scrape off the skin – no peeler required.

You can reserve the leftover solids and make more tea throughout the day, adding more tea leaves/bags and water as needed. Discard the solids at the end of the day.

To help the body better absorb the turmeric, add a few grinds of pepper when brewing the tea.

Early in 2013, I struggled with a strange allergic reaction that came out of the blue. After reading up a lot about natural solutions for allergies, I discovered rooibos tea. I decided to give this naturally sweet tea, long acclaimed for its healing properties, a shot. I started brewing rooibos with other superfoods like fresh turmeric, lemon, and ginger. While I still don't know the cause of my allergic reaction, I enjoyed this tea so much, it's something I now make on a regular basis. Add it to your own routine and let the healing powers begin!

Makes 1 litre

PREP TIME: 5 minutes • COOK TIME: 10 minutes

gluten-free, nut-free, oil-free, soy-free, refined sugar-free, grain-free

1. In a medium saucepan, combine the water, tea, lemon, turmeric, and ginger. Bring to a boil over medium-high heat, and then reduce the heat to medium-low and simmer for about 10 minutes, or longer, if you desire a stronger brew.

2. Pour the tea through a fine-mesh sieve placed over a bowl, stir in sweetener to taste, if desired, and serve immediately. Refrigerate the leftover tea and enjoy it chilled for a fun twist on classic iced tea.

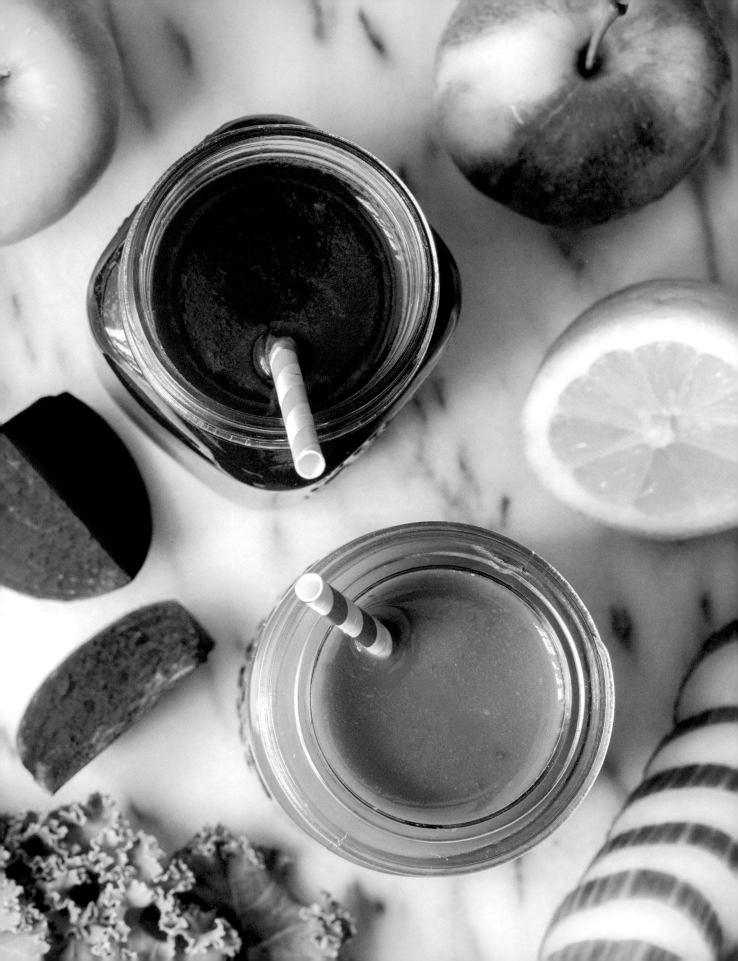

yogi juice

EVERYDAY GREEN JUICE:

Makes 500ml

1 seedless (English) cucumber, peeled and roughly chopped

4 small kale leaves, roughly chopped

1 sweet apple, cored and roughly chopped

1 ripe pear, cored and roughly chopped

1 to 2 tablespoons fresh lemon juice, to taste

BEET-UTIFUL POWER GLOW:

Makes 500 to 750ml

1 seedless (English) cucumber, peeled and roughly chopped

1 small to medium beet, peeled and roughly chopped

1 small to medium carrot, peeled and roughly chopped

1 to 2 tablespoons fresh lemon juice, to taste

1 small apple, cored and roughly chopped (optional)

I once owned a juicer and I loved having the ability to make fresh juice whenever I had a craving. I loathed the cleanup process that came afterward, however. Everyone says it's not that bad, but really, it is. Or maybe I'm just a lazy lump! When we moved to a place with a smaller kitchen, I donated my juicer to save space. Since then, I've discovered a method for making fresh juice at home with less cleanup; all you need is a blender and a straining bag (see page 24) or fine-mesh sieve. Here are a couple of my favourite juice blends to get you started. Keep in mind that these recipes can be made in a traditional juicer, too.

gluten-free, oil-free, raw/no-bake, sugar-free,
soy-free, grain-free, nut-free

1. In a high-speed blender, combine all of the ingredients with 125ml water and blend until smooth.

2. Place a straining bag (or fine-mesh sieve) over a large glass jar or bowl and slowly pour in the juice. Gently squeeze the straining bag to release the juice. If using a sieve, use a spoon to push through any remaining juice. Discard the pulp and enjoy!

3. Store any leftover juice in a canning jar in the refrigerator for 2 to 3 days.

Tips: If you want to keep the fibrous pulp in your drink, simply skip the straining and chug it back smoothie style – although be warned, it's very thick! Feel free to thin it out with more water.

If you aren't using a Vitamix or Blendtec blender, you might want to steam the beet before use.

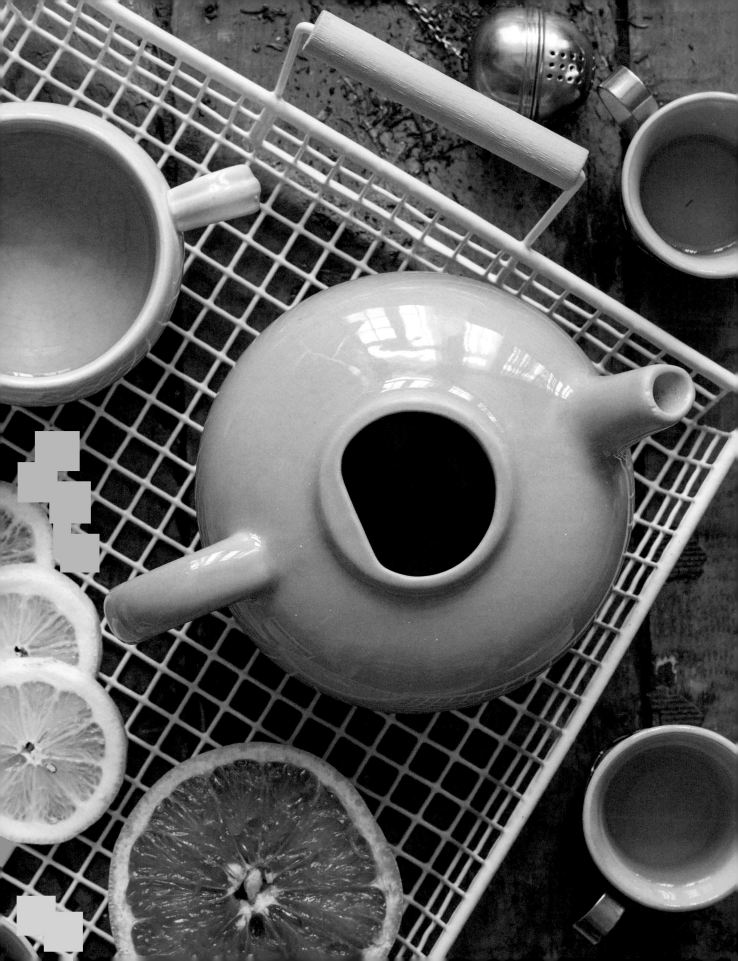

metabolism-boosting green citrus tea

1 green tea bag, or 1 teaspoon loose green tea

375ml boiling water

Juice of ½ grapefruit

Juice of ½ lemon

1½ to 3 teaspoons liquid sweetener, to taste

Very small pinch of cayenne pepper (optional)

This is an energizing green tea infused with grapefruit, lemon, and cayenne pepper – enjoy it any time your metabolism needs a little pick-me-up! It's one of my favorite ways to jump-start the day. If you'd like a chilled summer version, simply make a double batch at night and pop it in the fridge. You'll wake up to a chilled citrus tea you can enjoy all day long.

Makes 500ml

PREP TIME: 5 to 10 minutes

gluten-free, nut-free, oil-free, raw/no-bake, soy-free, grain-free, refined sugar free

1. Place the tea bag or loose tea (in a tea ball) in a very large mug (the mug should hold more than 500ml liquid). Let the boiling water sit for a few moments so it can come down in temperature slightly to avoid bitter green tea. Pour on the water and steep the tea for 3 minutes, then discard the bag or tea leaves.

2. Place a fine-mesh sieve over the mug and pour in the grapefruit and lemon juice to strain out any remaining pulp or seeds.

3. Stir in the sweetener and cayenne (if using), and immediately enjoy this metabolism-revving tea!

appetizers

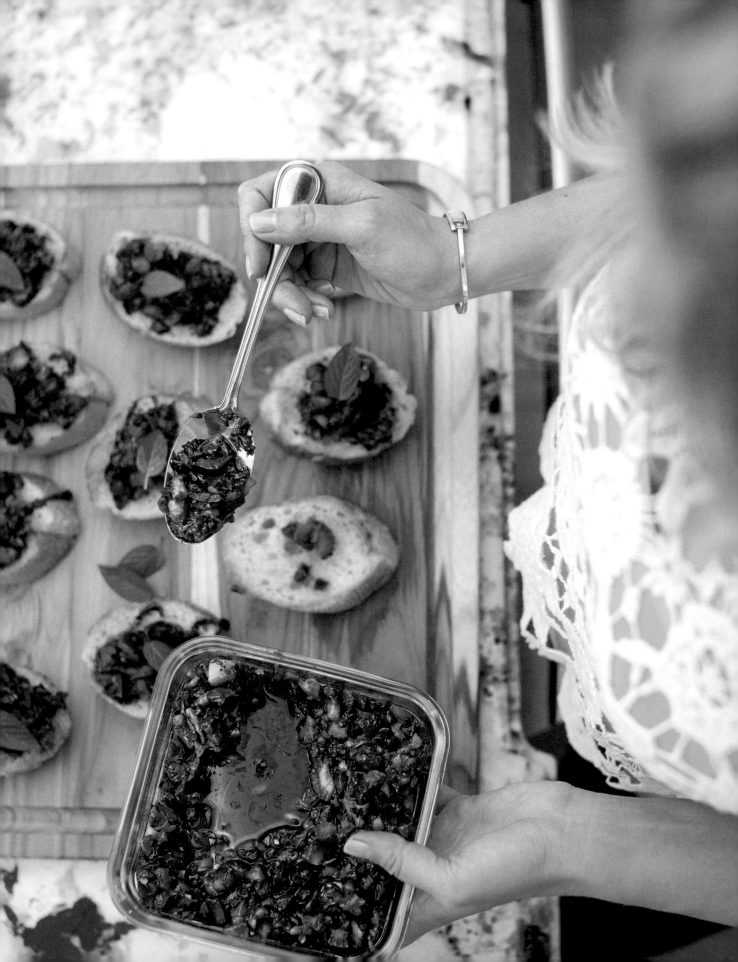

One of my favourite things to do is to entertain family and friends and treat them to all kinds of tasty vegan foods. It's a great way to introduce them to vegan cuisine, and many are often surprised by how much they enjoy animal-free recipes. The appetizers in this chapter are the ones I rely on the most for healthy finger foods. Not only will they please a crowd, but they leave all your guests feeling light and energized. No one wants to feel weighed down by greasy, heavy food at a party! My go-to party dip is my Life-Affirming Warm Nacho Dip (page 83); in case you can't tell by the name, we are pretty obsessed with it. On a chilly evening, it's the perfect dip to serve while watching the good ol' hockey game. If a summer appetizer is what you're looking for, try my Summertime Cherry-Basil Bruschetta (page 79), Glowing Strawberry-Mango Guacamole (page 81), or Oil-Free Baked Falafel Bites (page 95). It probably goes without saying, but many of these appetizers can be turned into mains. My husband and I have served Taco Fiesta Potato Crisps (page 85) and Oil-Free Baked Falafel Bites for dinner on several occasions. Okay, okay, we even had the Life-Affirming Warm Nacho Dip for dinner one night. Guilty as charged!

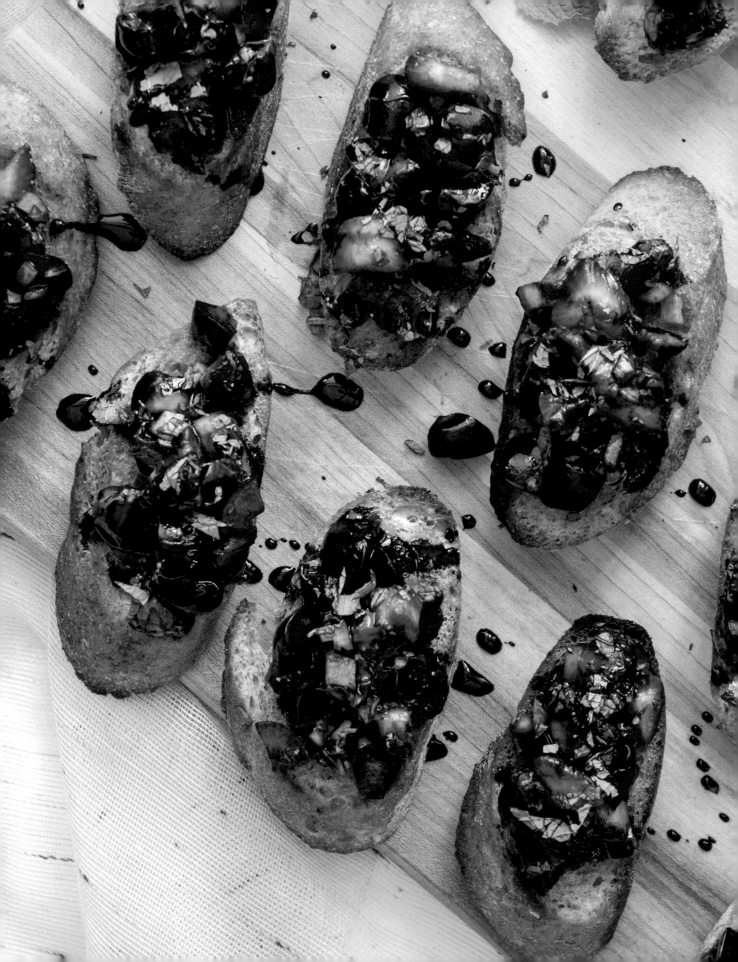

summertime cherry-basil bruschetta

225g fresh cherries, pitted and finely chopped

600g fresh strawberries, hulled and finely chopped

5g packed fresh basil leaves, minced

5g fresh mint leaves, minced

3 tablespoons finely chopped red onion

4 teaspoons balsamic vinegar

1 fresh baguette, sliced on an angle into 2.5cm pieces

2 tablespoons extra-virgin olive oil

1 recipe Balsamic Reduction (see page 297)

This is a showstopping, beautiful bruschetta, if I do say so myself. Elegant and classy, it'll have all your guests thinking you are a vegan version of Martha Stewart (only without the jail time, hopefully). If you've never had the combination of basil and berries before, you're in for a real treat!

Serves 2

PREP TIME: 20 minutes • COOK TIME: 5 to 7 minutes

nut-free, soy-free, sugar-free

1. Preheat the oven to 230°C (450°F).

2. In a large bowl, combine the cherries, strawberries, basil, mint, onion, and vinegar. Set the bruschetta topping aside for 10 to 15 minutes so the flavours can develop.

3. Brush one side of each piece of bread with oil and place them oil side down on a large rimmed baking sheet. Bake for 5 to 7 minutes, watching closely, until golden.

4. Spoon the bruschetta topping carefully onto the toasted bread. Drizzle each piece with some of the Balsamic Reduction and serve immediately.

Tip: Wear disposable plastic gloves when you make this recipe to keep your fingers stain-free and party ready.

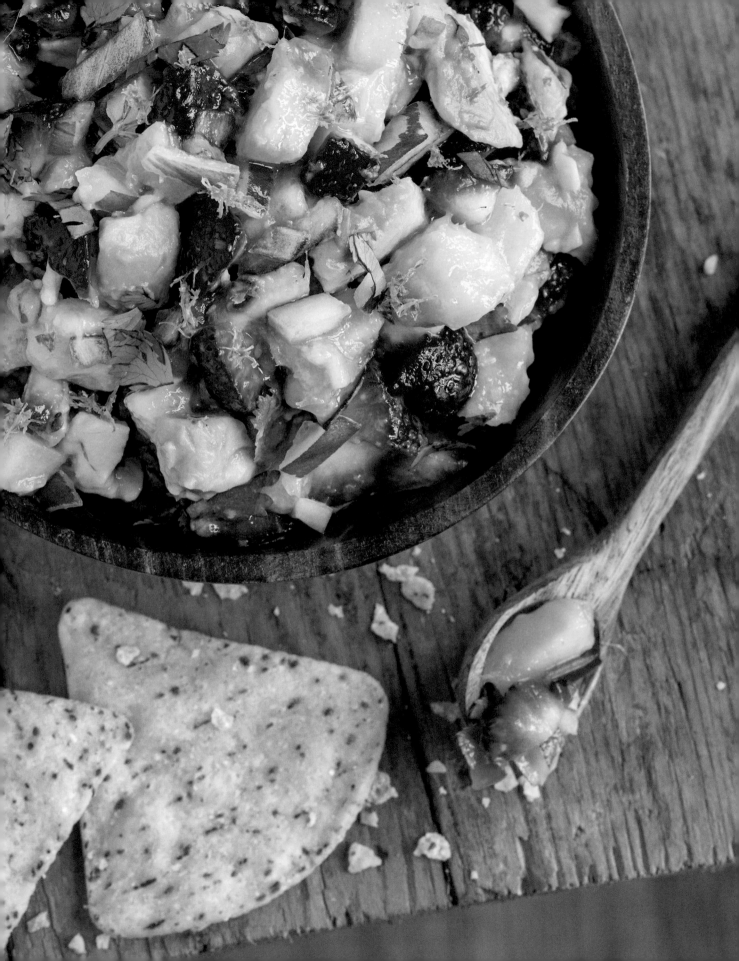

glowing strawberry-mango guacamole

2 medium avocados, pitted and roughly chopped

60g finely chopped red onion

1 fresh mango, pitted, peeled, and finely chopped

300g finely chopped hulled strawberries

5g fresh coriander leaves, roughly chopped (optional)

1 to 2 tablespoons fresh lime juice, to taste

Fine-grain sea salt

Corn chips, for serving

In this recipe, juicy, buttery mango and sweet strawberries liven up traditional guacamole. This bright, fruity guacamole never lasts long at a party because it leaves your guests feeling refreshed and energized. If you'd like to prepare this in advance, combine all of the ingredients except the avocado in an airtight container and keep it in the fridge. Just before serving, gently fold in the avocado and no one will be the wiser!

Makes 750ml

PREP TIME: 20 minutes

gluten-free, nut-free, oil-free, raw/no-bake,
soy-free, sugar-free, grain-free

1. In a medium bowl, gently mash the avocado, leaving some chunks for texture.

2. Rinse and drain the chopped onion in a strainer to wash off the sulfurous compounds. This makes the taste of the raw onion more pleasant. Fold the mango, strawberries, onion, and coriander (if using) into the avocado. Season with the lime juice and salt to taste.

3. Serve immediately with your favourite corn chips (or try my Spiced Toasted Pitta Chips, page 91). Avocado tends to spoil quickly, so leftovers won't keep for longer than 12 hours or so. One more reason to dig in!

Tip: For a spicy version, add 1 diced jalapeño to the mix. Omit the seeds for a just-a-bit-spicy version.

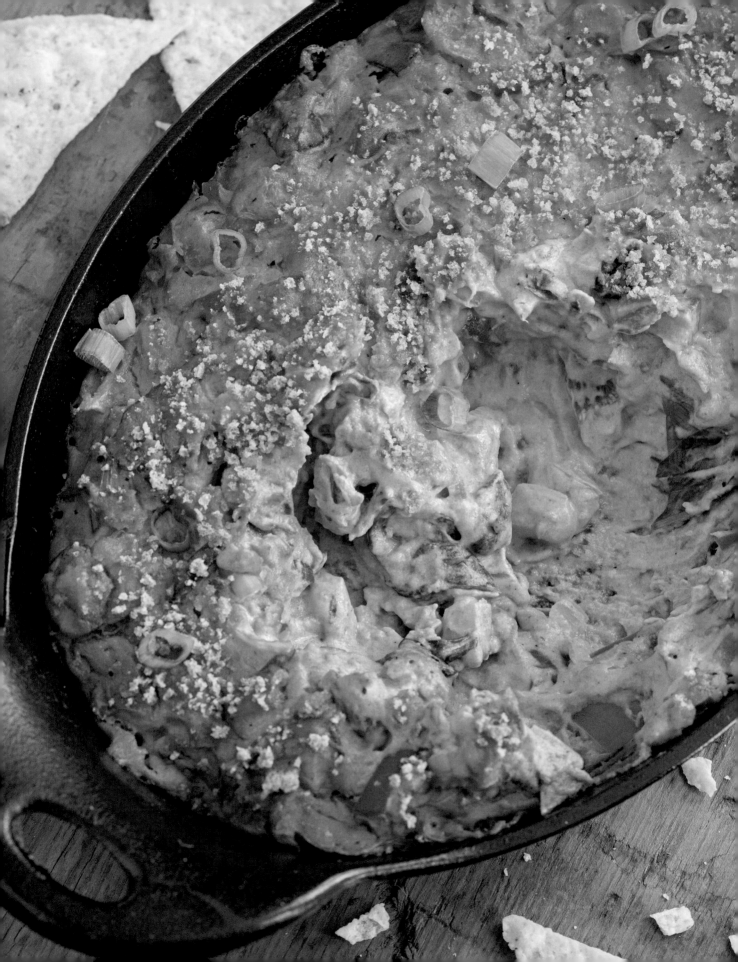

life-affirming warm nacho dip

FOR THE CHEESE SAUCE:

150g raw cashews

150g peeled and chopped carrots

2 tablespoons nutritional yeast

2 tablespoons fresh lemon juice

1 large clove garlic

1¼ teaspoons fine-grain sea salt

¾ teaspoon chilli powder

½ teaspoon onion powder

¼ to ½ teaspoon cayenne pepper, to taste (optional)

FOR THE DIP:

250ml chunky marinara sauce

150g finely chopped sweet onion

2 to 3 handfuls of baby spinach roughly chopped

30g crushed corn chips or breadcrumbs

1 to 2 green onions, finely sliced, for serving (optional)

Tortilla chips or Spiced Toasted Pitta Chips (see page 91), for serving

You'd never know there isn't a lick of dairy or oil hiding in this mouthwatering hot-out-of-the-oven dip! This dish is always a crowd-pleaser. It's best when hot, so serve it on a plate warmer or pot holder so it stays warm for as long as possible. I like to bake it in a cast-iron dish, which keeps it warm for almost an hour.

Serves 8

PREP TIME: 25 to 30 minutes, plus soaking time

COOK TIME: 25 to 30 minutes

gluten-free option, oil-free, soy-free, sugar-free, grain-free

1. Make the Cheese Sauce: Place the cashews in a medium bowl and add water to cover. Set aside to soak for at least 2 hours, or overnight if you have the time. Drain and rinse the soaked cashews.

2. Preheat the oven to 200°C (400°F). Lightly grease a 2-litre cast-iron pan or casserole dish.

3. Place the carrots in a small saucepan and add water to cover. Bring the water to a boil and cook the carrots for 5 minutes, or until just fork-tender. Drain. You can also steam the carrots, if desired.

4. In a blender, combine the soaked and drained cashews, cooked carrots, nutritional yeast, lemon juice, garlic, salt, chilli powder, onion powder, cayenne (if using), and 150ml water and blend until silky smooth, adding a splash of extra water if needed. Pour the sauce into a large bowl.

5. Make the Dip: Stir the marinara sauce, onion, and spinach into the Cheese Sauce until fully combined. Spoon the sauce into the prepared dish and smooth out, and sprinkle the top evenly with the crushed corn chips.

6. Bake for 25 to 30 minutes, uncovered, watching closely towards the end of the cooking time to make sure the corn chip topping doesn't burn. Garnish with sliced green onion, if desired. Serve immediately with tortilla chips or Spiced Toasted Pitta Chips.

7. Reheat any leftovers in the oven at 200°C (400°F) for 10 to 20 minutes, or until heated through. Store the dip in an airtight container in the fridge for 3 to 5 days.

Tip: For a gluten-free option, use crushed corn chips and corn tortilla chips for serving.

taco fiesta potato crisps

FOR THE POTATO CRISPS:
2 russet potatoes, unpeeled, sliced into 6mm rounds

1 tablespoon grapeseed oil

Fine-grain sea salt and freshly ground black pepper

FOR THE WALNUT TACO MEAT:
100g walnuts, toasted, if preferred

1 tablespoon olive oil

1½ teaspoons chilli powder

½ teaspoon ground cumin

¼ teaspoon fine-grain sea salt

⅛ teaspoon cayenne pepper

TO ASSEMBLE:
1 recipe Cashew Sour Cream (see page 281)

125 to 175ml salsa

2 to 3 green onions, thinly sliced

Freshly ground black pepper

Quite possibly the ultimate party finger food, these potato taco crisps are almost too good to share. I speak from experience; my husband and I once polished off an entire batch before our friends even made it to the party! It was a bit embarrassing explaining that we had demolished their appetizer. Oops. The base is made of roasted potato slices that are topped with a crunchy Walnut Taco Meat, Cashew Sour Cream, and salsa. If you don't have time to layer everything individually, try plating the potato crisps on a large platter and layer everything all at once. The walnut taco meat and Cashew Sour Cream can be made a day or two in advance to save some time. The crisps also make a fun – and definitely kid-approved – dinner.

Makes 28 to 30 crisps
PREP TIME: 25 to 30 minutes • COOK TIME: 35 minutes
gluten-free, soy-free, sugar-free, grain-free

1. Make the Potato Crisps: Preheat the oven to 220°C (425°F). Line a large rimmed baking sheet with parchment paper. Place the potato slices in a single layer on the baking sheet and drizzle them with the oil. Rub the potatoes to disperse the oil evenly. Sprinkle the potatoes generously with salt and pepper.

2. Roast the potatoes for 30 to 35 minutes, flipping them once halfway through, until tender and lightly browned. Allow the potatoes to cool for 5 minutes before assembling.

3. Make the Walnut Taco Meat: In a mini food processor, combine the walnuts, oil, chilli powder, cumin, salt, and cayenne and process into a fine crumble. (You can also chop and mix the ingredients by hand, if preferred.) Set aside.

4. To assemble, top each potato slice with 1 teaspoon of the Cashew Sour Cream, followed by about 1 teaspoon each of the walnut taco

meat, salsa, and green onions, in that order. Garnish with pepper. Serve immediately, while still warm.

Tip: Instead of potatoes, try serving the toppings on lettuce cups, or pair them with tortilla chips for a satisfying vegan nacho plate.

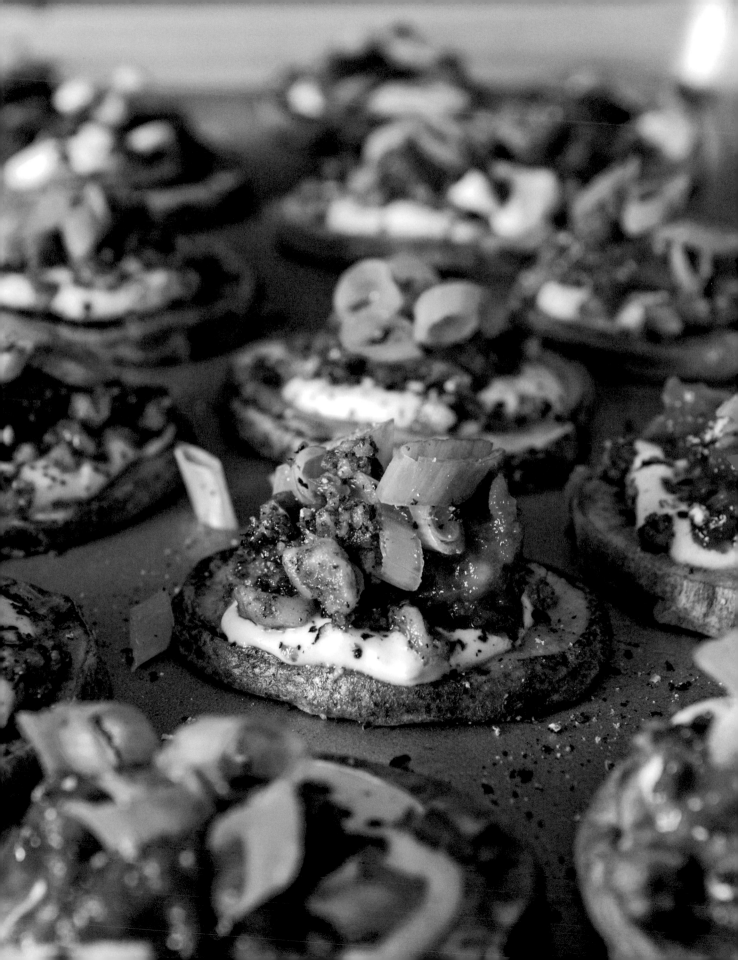

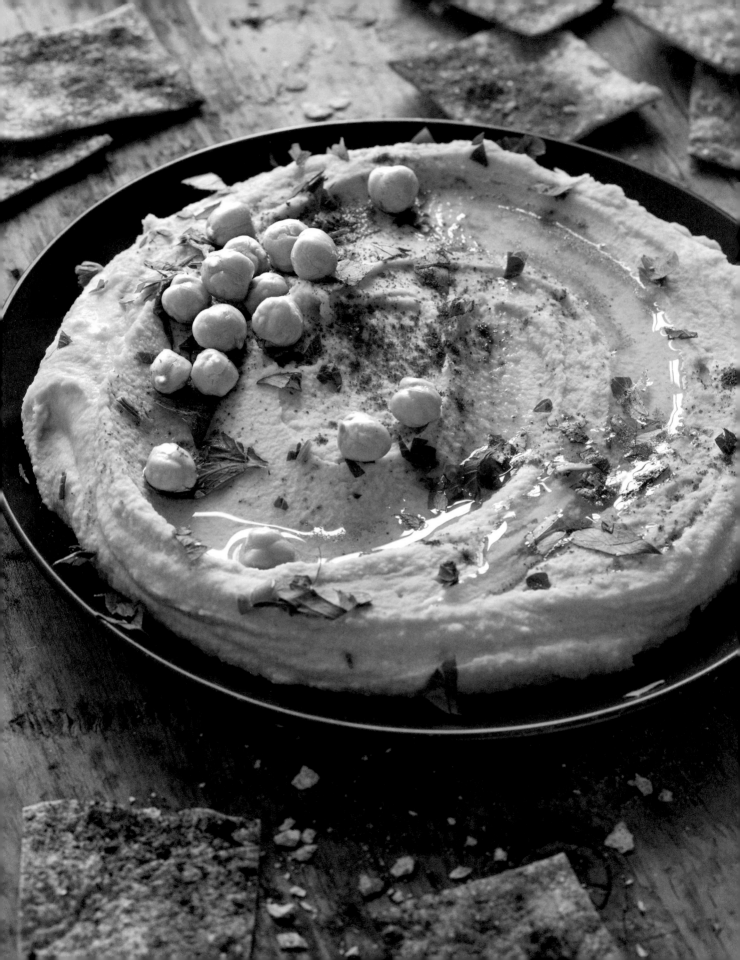

classic hummus

600g cooked chickpeas (from 200g dry chickpeas or two 425g cans)

1 large or 2 small cloves garlic

75ml tahini

60ml fresh lemon juice (from about 1 lemon), or to taste

1 teaspoon fine-grain sea salt, or to taste

5 to 10 drops hot sauce (optional)

Extra-virgin olive oil, paprika, and minced parsley, for serving

Spiced Toasted Pitta Chips (see page 91), for serving

I fussed and fussed with testing all different kinds of hummus flavours for this book. You name it, I probably tried it. Despite my best efforts, I kept coming back to this classic hummus recipe. The truth is, if it ain't broke, don't fix it! Throughout my hummus-testing process, I discovered two secrets that will take your hummus from tasty to prize-worthy. The first tip involves cooking the chickpeas from scratch. In a side-by-side taste test of freshly cooked versus canned beans, I couldn't believe the difference in flavour. While I have no problem using canned chickpeas in a pinch, fresh-cooked beans just taste so much better. Second, if you have fifteen extra minutes (and a partner you can bribe to help), pop the skin off the chickpeas before adding them to the processor. You'll be rewarded with ultra-smooth hummus that rivals any store-bought version.

Makes 625ml

PREP TIME: 10 to 20 minutes

gluten-free, nut-free, soy-free, sugar-free, raw/no-bake, grain-free

1. Rinse and drain the chickpeas. If you have time, remove the skins: Squeeze a chickpea between your forefinger and thumb and push to pop off the skin. Discard the skins, and set aside a handful of chickpeas for serving.

2. With the food processor running, add the garlic to mince.

3. Add the chickpeas, tahini, lemon juice, salt, and hot sauce (if using), and process until combined, adjusting the quantities as needed to taste. Add 4 to 6 tablespoons water to reach the desired consistency. Process until smooth, scraping down the bowl as needed. (I like to let my processor run for at least a couple of minutes.)

4. Transfer the hummus to a serving bowl and top with a drizzle of

olive oil, the reserved chickpeas, a sprinkle of paprika, and minced parsley. Serve with Spiced Toasted Pitta Chips, if desired.

Tips: Homemade hummus has a tendency to thicken when chilled. To thin it out, simply add a splash of olive oil or water and stir to combine. Homemade hummus will keep in an airtight container in the fridge for at least 1 week.

For how to cook chickpeas from scratch, see page 14.

spiced toasted pitta chips

2 pittas or tortillas

2 teaspoons extra-virgin olive oil

½ teaspoon garlic powder

½ teaspoon ground cumin

½ teaspoon paprika

¼ teaspoon fine-grain sea salt

I love to season pitta bread or tortillas with a bit of garlic powder, cumin, and paprika and bake it in the oven until crisp. After toasting in the oven, you're left with scrumptious, crunchy pitta chips that make a lovely pair with Classic Hummus (page 89). Be warned – they won't last long!

Makes about 40 chips

PREP TIME: 5 minutes • COOK TIME: 7 to 9 minutes

nut-free, soy-free, sugar-free

1. Preheat the oven to 200°C (400°F).

2. With kitchen shears, cut the pittas into wedges about the size of tortilla chips. Arrange them in a single layer on a large rimmed baking sheet.

3. With a pastry brush, spread the oil on the pitta wedges and sprinkle them generously with the garlic powder, cumin, paprika, and salt.

4. Bake for 7 to 9 minutes, or until golden. Remove from the oven and let cool. The chips will firm up after about 5 to 10 minutes of cooling.

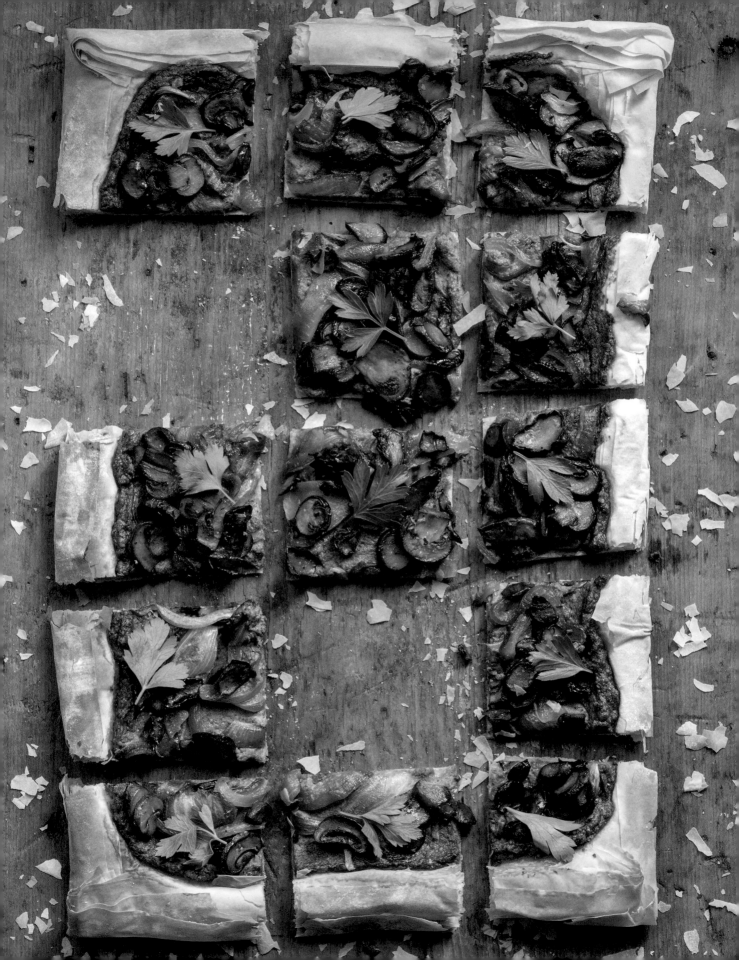

mushroom-walnut pesto tart

FOR THE SAUTÉED MUSHROOMS AND ONIONS:

2 tablespoons extra-virgin olive oil

420g sliced cremini mushrooms

1 medium red onion, peeled and halved lengthwise and sliced into thin half-moons

FOR THE WALNUT PESTO:

1 large clove garlic

60g toasted walnuts

20g loosely packed fresh parsley, large stems removed

60ml extra-virgin olive oil

½ to ¾ teaspoon fine-grain sea salt, to taste

½ teaspoon freshly ground black pepper

TO ASSEMBLE:

7 to 8 sheets frozen filo pastry, thawed

Olive oil, for brushing the dough

Handful of fresh parsley leaves (optional)

This pesto tart took home first prize in a Mushroom Canada competition a few years ago. Not only is it one of my favourite appetizer recipes, but many *Oh She Glows* readers have tried this award winner to great success. It takes a bit of time to prepare, but the wait is worth it once you sink your teeth into your first crispy, savoury bite. If you don't want to make a filo tart, you can simply spread the pesto onto crostini, or try tossing it with pasta for an elegant dinner. The sky's the limit, dear mushroom fan! Be sure to thaw the filo pastry overnight so it's ready when you make the tart.

Serves 6 to 8

PREP TIME: 45 minutes • COOK TIME: 26 to 32 minutes

soy-free, sugar-free

1. Preheat the oven to 180°C (350°F). Line a large rimmed baking sheet with parchment paper.

2. Make the Sautéed Mushrooms and Onions: In a large frying pan, heat 1 tablespoon of the oil over a medium-high heat. Add the mushrooms and sauté until the liquid released by the mushrooms has evaporated and the mushrooms are tender, 15 to 25 minutes. Set aside.

3. Meanwhile, in another large frying pan, heat the remaining 1 tablespoon oil over medium-low heat. Add the onion and sauté, stirring often, until soft and translucent, about 20 minutes. Set aside.

4. Make the Walnut Pesto: In a food processor, pulse the garlic to finely chop it. Add the walnuts, parsley, oil, salt, pepper, 70g of the sautéed mushrooms, and 2 tablespoons of water and process until smooth, stopping to scrape down the bowl as necessary.

5. Assemble the Tart: Place 1 sheet of filo pastry on the prepared baking sheet and lightly spray it with oil (or brush on some oil with

a pastry brush). Place another sheet of filo directly on top of the first and spray or brush it with oil. Repeat with the remaining 5 to 6 sheets of pastry. Fold the edges in by 2.5cm on all sides to create a border and press to adhere. (See photo on page 92.) If it's not sticking, lightly spray (or brush) the filo with oil and try again. With a fork, poke a few holes into the pastry to allow steam to escape during cooking.

6. Gently spread the Walnut Pesto in an even layer over the surface, keeping it within the folded borders. Distribute the remaining sautéed mushrooms and all of the sautéed onion evenly over the pesto.

7. Bake the tart for 26 to 32 minutes, or until it is lightly golden and crispy to the touch. If you'd like nice golden edges on the tart, grill it for 1 to 2 minutes after baking, watching it closely to make sure it doesn't burn.

8. Cool the tart for 5 minutes before slicing it with a pizza slicer. Garnish with fresh parsley, if desired, and serve immediately.

Tip: To save time, buy pre-sliced mushrooms. Our little secret!

oil-free baked falafel bites

FOR THE FALAFEL:

3 cloves garlic

50g red onion

10g packed fresh coriander leaves

10g packed fresh parsley leaves

1 425g can chickpeas, drained and rinsed

2 tablespoons ground flaxseed

25g plus 6 tablespoons spelt breadcrumbs or Sprouted-Grain Breadcrumbs (see page 279)

½ teaspoon ground cumin

½ teaspoon fine-grain sea salt

FOR THE TOMATO-CUCUMBER SALSA:

300g grape tomatoes

25g red onions

5g fresh coriander

1 tablespoon fresh lime juice

75g diced cucumber

Fine-grain sea salt

TO ASSEMBLE:

Leaves from 1 head of Bibb, Boston, or romaine lettuce

Lemon-Tahini Dressing (see page 284)

This lightened-up take on traditional falafel will leave you feeling light and energized, and not at all weighed down. Rather than deep-frying the falafel, I've rolled them in crunchy whole grain spelt breadcrumbs and then baked them in the oven. The breadcrumbs give the falafel the nice crunch of a deep-fried version, but without all the oil and grease. Now that's something to smile about!

Makes 22 bite-size falafel

PREP TIME: 30 minutes • COOK TIME: 30 minutes

nut-free, soy-free, sugar-free

1. Make the Falafel: Preheat the oven to 200°C (400°F). Line a large rimmed baking sheet with parchment paper.

2. In a food processor, pulse the garlic to finely chop it. Add the onion, coriander, and parsley and process until minced. Add the chickpeas and process until the mixture forms a coarse dough and holds together when pressed between your fingers.

3. Transfer the mixture to a large bowl and stir in the flaxseed, 25g of the breadcrumbs, cumin, and salt until combined.

4. Shape the mixture into small patties, using about 1 tablespoon dough for each and pressing each firmly to hold its shape. Repeat until you have used all of the chickpea mixture.

5. With a pastry brush, brush a few drops of water onto each patty. One at a time, roll the patties in the remaining 6 tablespoons of breadcrumbs, pressing down on each side so the breadcrumbs stick. (The crumbs don't tend to stick that well, so you have to make an effort to press them in.) Repeat until all of the patties have been coated. Place onto a prepared baking sheet.

6. Bake the falafel until golden brown, about 30 minutes, flipping once halfway through the baking time.

7. Make the Tomato-Cucumber Salsa: In a food processor, combine the tomatoes, onion, coriander, and lime juice and process until roughly chopped. Stir in the diced cucumber and salt to taste.

8. To assemble, arrange the lettuce leaves in a single layer on a serving tray. Place 1 falafel in the centre of each lettuce leaf. Top with some of the Tomato-Cucumber Salsa and a drizzle of Lemon-Tahini Dressing.

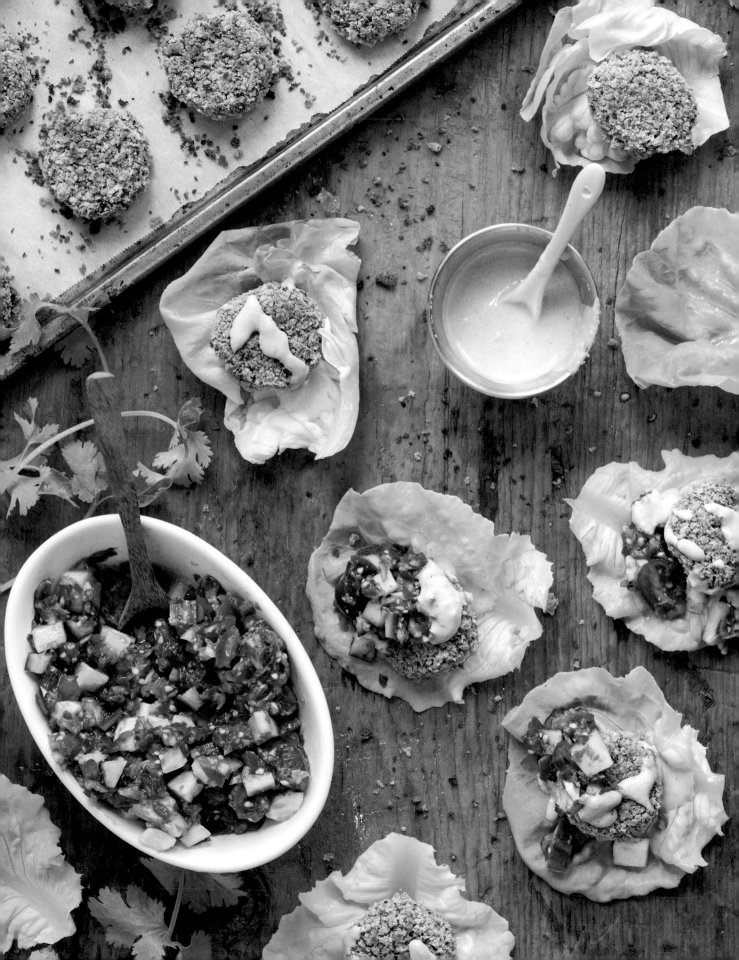

salads

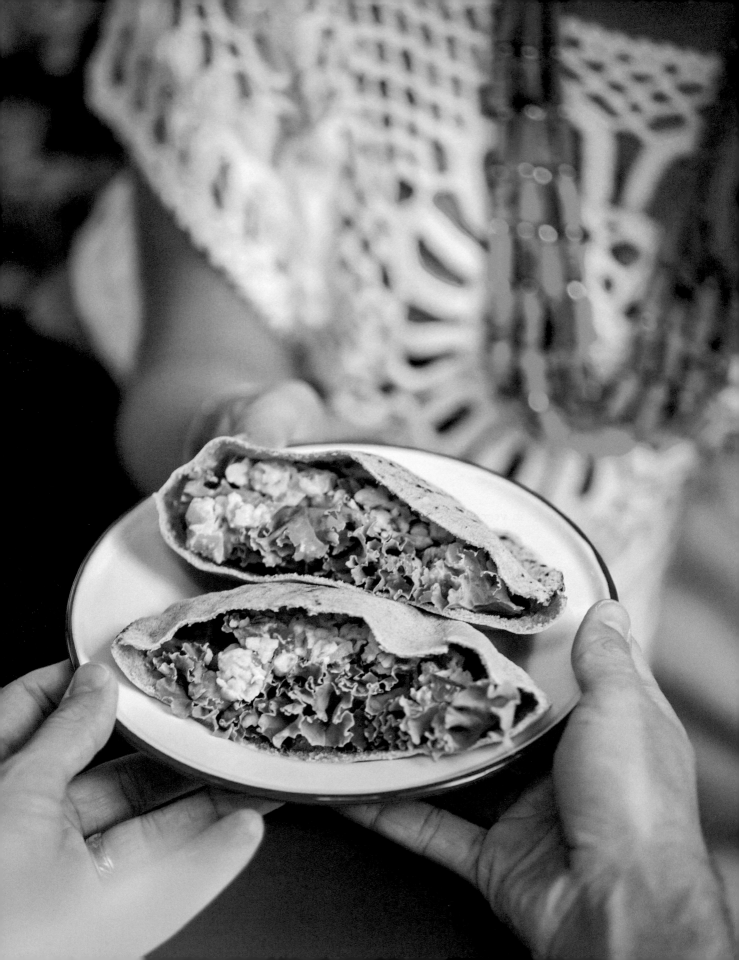

I'm sure it sounds like a cliché coming from a vegan, but this is the chapter that excites me the most. I've suffered through one too many plain-Jane lettuce and tomato salads in my day, so my goal when creating salad recipes is to bust the stereotype that salads are boring, diet food. Au contraire! My salads are anything but dull and boring, and I take great pride in creating hearty, drool-worthy delights. Packed with plant-based protein, crispy fresh vegetables, and heart-healthy dressings, you'll wonder how you ever got into a salad rut in the first place. From my Creamy Avocado-Potato Salad (page 107) to Chakra Caesar Salad (page 109), there's a salad for whatever mood you're in. Sharpen that knife, whip out the chopping board, and get ready to feel the glow!

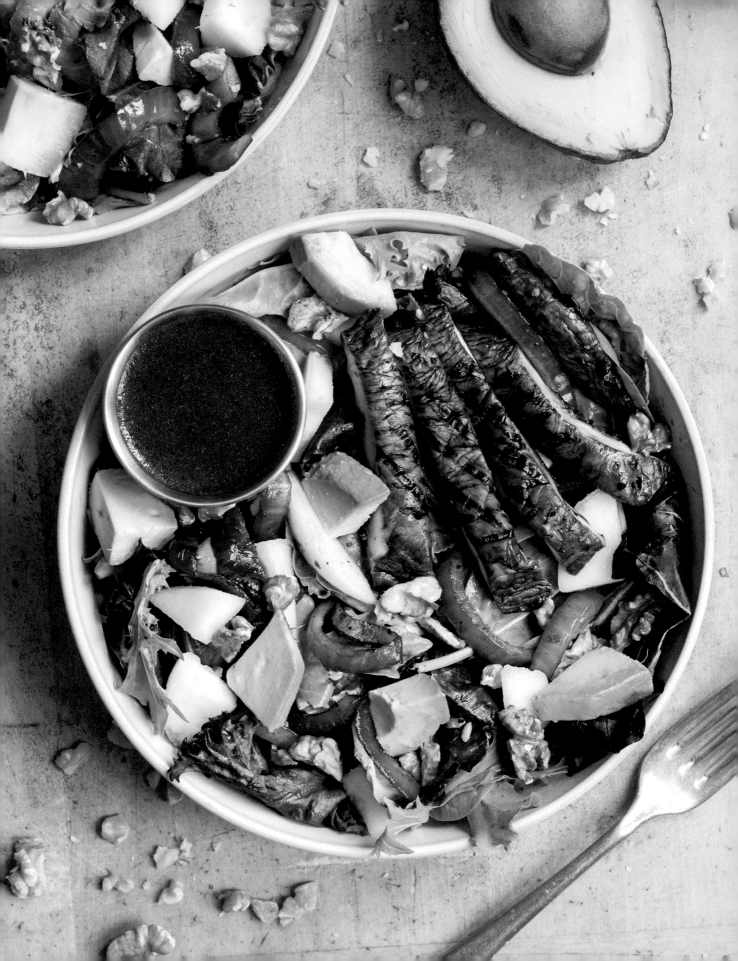

walnut, avocado & pear salad with marinated portobello caps & red onion

2 large portobello mushrooms

½ red onion, thinly sliced

1 recipe Effortless Anytime Balsamic Vinaigrette (see page 283)

142g mixed greens

2 ripe pears, peeled, cored, and chopped

1 avocado, pitted and chopped

40g walnuts, toasted

This salad was inspired by a dish at a local restaurant where my girlfriends and I meet for lunch once a month. With buttery pear slices, grilled marinated red onion, portobello mushrooms, toasted walnuts, and creamy avocado, it's a delicious mix of my favourite flavours and textures, and it's filling, too. Each portobello mushroom packs in around 6 to 8 grams protein, so add one or two and you have yourself a protein-packed salad that will go the distance.

Serves 2

PREP TIME: 15 to 20 minutes • COOK TIME: 8 to 10 minutes

gluten-free, soy-free, refined sugar-free, grain-free

1. Gently rub the outside of the mushrooms with a damp towel to remove any debris. Remove the stems by twisting the stem until it pops off; discard it or freeze for another use, such as a stir-fry. With a small spoon, scrape out and discard the black gills.

2. In a large bowl, combine the mushroom caps, onion, and half of the balsamic vinaigrette and toss until fully coated. Marinate the mushrooms and onion for 20 to 30 minutes, tossing every 5 to 10 minutes.

3. Heat a grill pan over a medium-high heat. Place the mushroom caps and onion on the pan and grill for 3 to 5 minutes per side, until grill marks appear and the vegetables are tender. Reduce the heat if necessary. Remove the pan from the heat and set aside until the mushroom caps are cool enough to handle, then slice the mushroom caps into long strips.

4. For each salad, place a few handfuls of mixed greens in a large bowl and top with half of the chopped pear, avocado, walnuts, and grilled mushrooms and onion. Drizzle the salad with some of the remaining balsamic vinaigrette and enjoy!

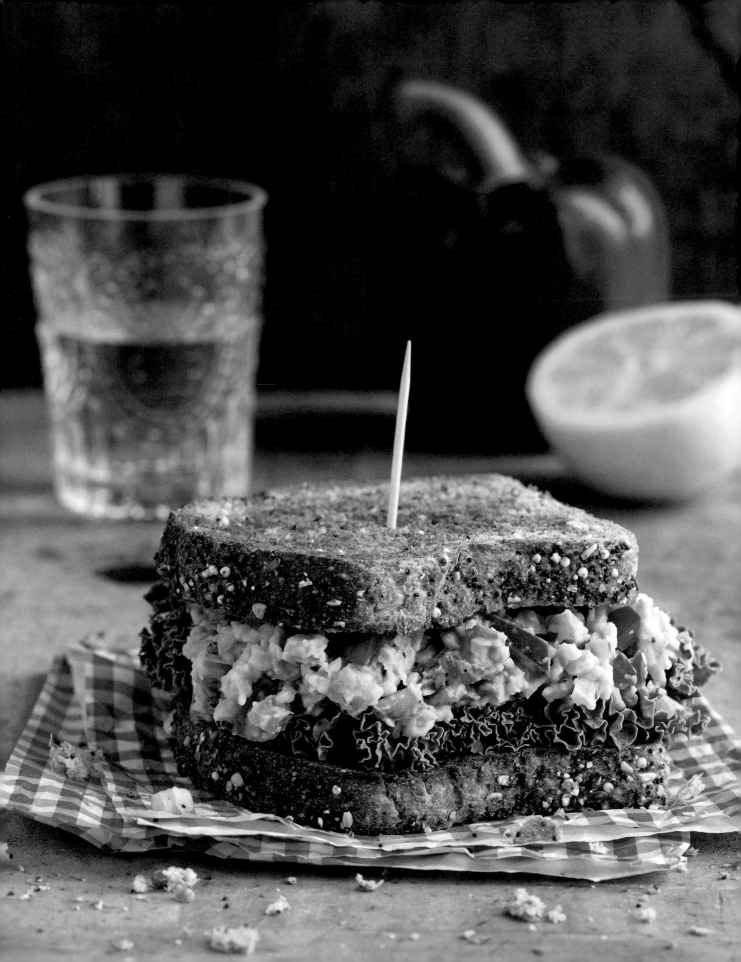

perfected chickpea salad sandwich

1 425g can chickpeas, drained and rinsed

2 stalks celery, finely chopped

3 green onions, thinly sliced

40g finely chopped dill pickle

40g finely chopped red bell pepper

2 to 3 tablespoons store-bought or homemade vegan mayonnaise (see page 278)

1 clove garlic, minced

1½ teaspoons yellow mustard

2 teaspoons minced fresh dill (optional)

1½ to 3 teaspoons fresh lemon juice, to taste

¼ teaspoon fine-grain sea salt, or to taste

Freshly ground black pepper

Toasted bread, crackers, tortillas, or lettuce, for serving

Tip: If you'd like a soy-free version of this salad, be sure to use soy-free vegan mayonnaise. Veganaise makes a great option.

Before I became a vegan, I used to prepare canned flaked chicken regularly. This chickpea salad is my alternative to the chicken salad sandwiches of my youth. I must say, this version blows the former out of the park! The mashed chickpeas create a texture very similar to flaked chicken and the sauce gets a boost from a creamy eggless mayonnaise. I've also added a hefty amount of vegetables like celery, green onion, pickles, and bell peppers to give it a great crunch and loads of fibre. Serve this salad in pieces of Boston or Bibb lettuce, in a wrap or sandwich, or on crackers. If you have a picnic or road trip coming up, you'll be happy to know that it packs well, too.

Serves 3

PREP TIME: 15 minutes

gluten-free, nut-free, raw/no-bake, sugar-free,
grain-free, soy-free option

1. In a large bowl, mash the chickpeas with a potato masher until flaky in texture.

2. Stir in the celery, green onions, pickles, bell peppers, mayonnaise, and garlic until combined.

3. Stir in the mustard and dill (if using) and season with the lemon juice, salt, and black pepper, adjusting the quantities to taste.

4. Serve with toasted bread, on crackers, in a tortilla or lettuce wrap, or on top of a basic leafy green salad.

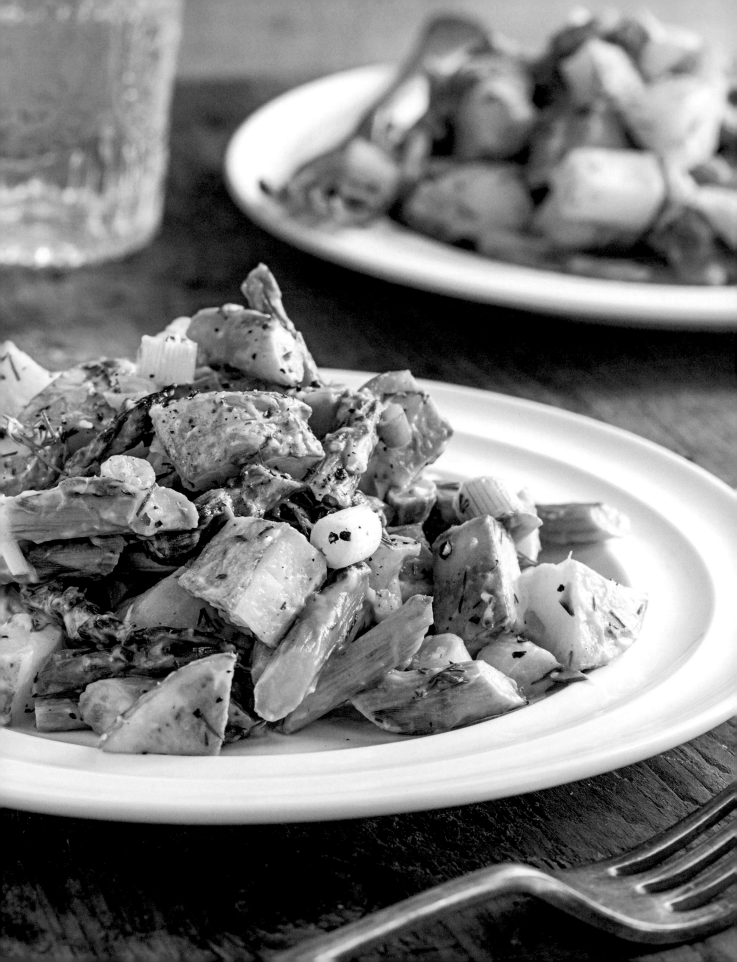

creamy avocado-potato salad

675 to 900g yellow potatoes, chopped into 1cm cubes

3 teaspoons extra-virgin olive oil

½ teaspoon fine-grain sea salt

¼ teaspoon freshly ground black pepper

1 bunch asparagus, woody ends broken off, stalks chopped into 2.5cm pieces

50g chopped green onions

FOR THE DRESSING:
150g avocado

2 tablespoons minced fresh dill

4 teaspoons fresh lemon juice

1 green onion, roughly chopped

¼ teaspoon fine-grain sea salt, or to taste, plus more for serving

Freshly ground black pepper

This recipe blends avocado with fresh dill, green onion, and lemon juice to create a tangy, creamy dressing for roasted potatoes and asparagus. I promise you will never see potato salad in the same way ever again! Traditional potato salads tend to call for boiled potatoes, but I like to use crispy roasted potatoes to give my potato salads a fantastic, mush-free texture. Try it and see the difference for yourself.

Serves 3

PREP TIME: 25 minutes

COOK TIME: 30 to 35 minutes

gluten-free, nut-free, soy-free, sugar-free, grain-free

1. Preheat the oven to 220°C (425°F). Line two rimmed baking sheets with parchment paper.

2. Spread the potatoes in an even layer on one of the prepared baking sheets and drizzle them with 1½ teaspoons of the oil. Season with half of the salt and pepper. Spread the asparagus on the second baking sheet and drizzle with the remaining 1½ teaspoons oil. Season with the remaining salt and pepper.

3. Roast the potatoes for 15 minutes, flip them over, and then roast them for 15 to 20 minutes more, until golden and fork-tender. During the last 15 minutes of roasting the potatoes, place the asparagus in the oven and roast for 9 to 12 minutes, until tender. Transfer the roasted potatoes and asparagus to a large bowl and stir in the green onions.

4. Make the Dressing: In a mini food processor, combine the avocado, dill, lemon juice, green onion, salt, pepper, to taste, and 60ml water and process until smooth.

5. Add the dressing to the bowl with the potatoes and asparagus and stir until combined. Season with salt and pepper to taste and serve immediately. The salad is also good chilled and will keep in an airtight container in the refrigerator for a couple of days.

chakra caesar salad
with nutty herb croutons

FOR THE DRESSING:

70g whole raw almonds

1 whole head garlic, for roasting, plus ½ clove garlic, minced (optional)

60ml extra-virgin olive oil

4 teaspoons fresh lemon juice

1 teaspoon Dijon mustard

¼ to ½ teaspoon fine-grain sea salt, to taste

¼ teaspoon dry mustard

½ teaspoon freshly ground black pepper

2 heads romaine lettuce, chopped, or a mix of romaine and destemmed torn kale leaves

1 recipe Nutty Herb Croutons (see page 296)

As a child, I grew up helping my dad prepare his 'famous' Caesar salad during every holiday. He'd wash multiple heads of romaine lettuce over the sink while my sister and I lined up at the drying station, meticulously dabbing each leaf with heaps of paper towel. You see, someone who makes a famous Caesar salad like my dad is suspicious of salad spinners and insists that the lettuce must be *hand-dried* to ensure that *every last drop* of water is soaked up. Even though I detested this long drying process, I knew I'd be enjoying his salad soon enough. I guess it comes as no surprise that I wanted to create my own version of Caesar salad for this book, one that would stand up to his version. Sorry, Dad, but I think this salad is even better, and you don't need the raw eggs! In my version, soaked raw almonds create the creamy, healthy base in place of raw eggs or mayonnaise. Roasted garlic makes the dressing creamier and a little more mellow. Oh, and don't worry: I highly recommend using a salad spinner if you have one. Let's be real.

*Makes 175ml dressing
(enough for 4 to 6 servings)*

PREP TIME: 20 minutes • COOK TIME: 35 to 40 minutes

gluten-free, soy-free, sugar-free, grain-free

1. Make the Dressing: Place the almonds in a bowl and add enough water to cover. Soak the almonds for at least 12 hours, or overnight. Drain and rinse the almonds. Pop off the skins by pressing the base of each almond between your thumb and forefinger. (Removing the skins yields a smoother dressing, but it's not absolutely essential.)

2. Preheat the oven to 220°C (425°F).

3. Cut off the top of the garlic head so all of the raw cloves are exposed. Remove any loose skin. Wrap the head in foil and place it

on a baking sheet. Roast the garlic for 35 to 40 minutes, or until the cloves are soft and golden. Cool for 10 to 15 minutes, until cold enough to handle. Remove the foil and squeeze the garlic cloves out of their skins and into a food processor.

4. Add the soaked almonds, oil, lemon juice, Dijon mustard, salt, dry mustard, pepper, and 60ml water to the food processor and process until smooth, stopping to scrape down the bowl as needed. Taste and add more salt and pepper as needed. Add the minced raw garlic if you'd like the dressing to have a more intense garlic flavour – otherwise, leave it out.

5. Place the lettuce in a large salad bowl and pour your desired amount of dressing on top. Toss until fully coated. Sprinkle the Nutty Herb Croutons over the salad just before serving.

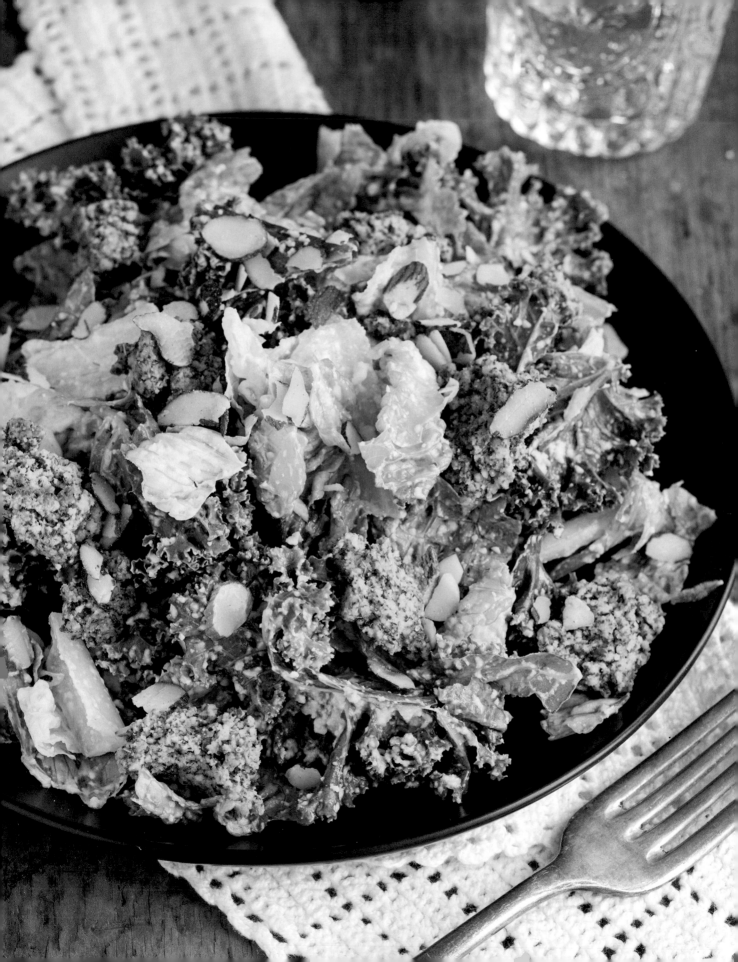

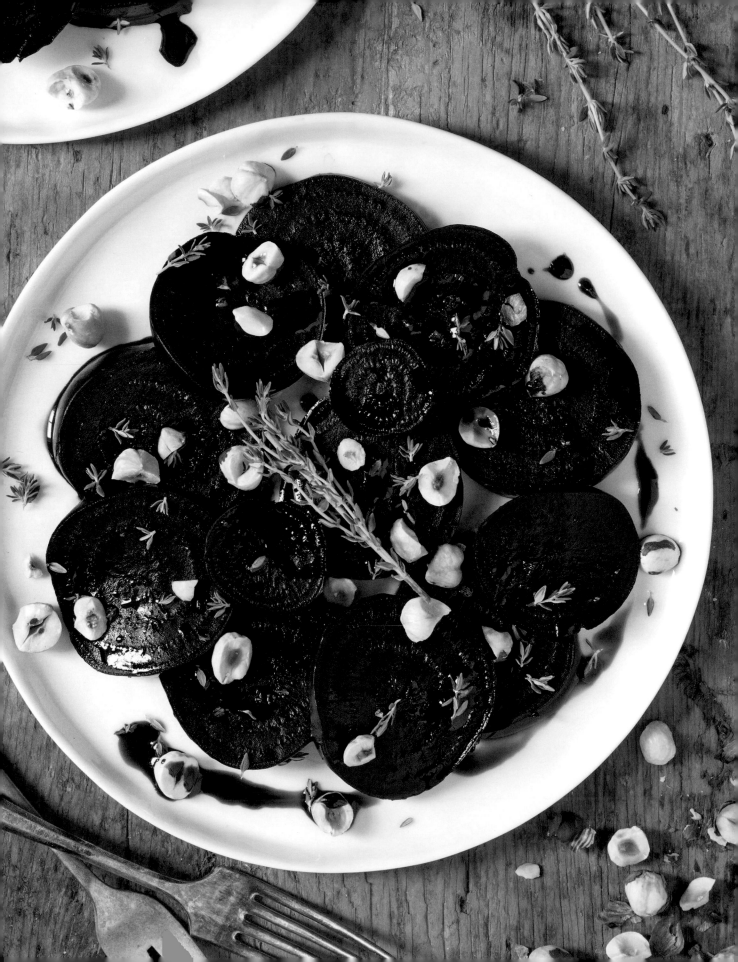

roasted beet salad with hazelnuts, thyme & balsamic reduction

5 to 6 medium beets, trimmed

75g hazelnuts, toasted

3 to 4 tablespoons Balsamic Reduction (see page 297)

1 tablespoon roasted hazelnut oil or extra-virgin olive oil

6 to 8 sprigs fresh thyme

This salad is inspired by Millennium, one of my favorite vegan restaurants in San Francisco. Their simple, yet highly nutritious, roasted beet salad is so flavourful and satisfying, when I tried it, I knew I had to create something similar at home. Enjoy this comforting salad as a lovely starter to any fall or winter meal.

Serves 3

PREP TIME: 20 to 25 minutes

COOK TIME: 1 hour to 1 hour and 30 minutes

gluten-free, soy-free, sugar-free, grain-free

1. Preheat the oven to 200°C (400°F).

2. Wrap each beet individually in a piece of foil and place them on a baking sheet. Roast the beets for 45 to 90 minutes, depending on the size of the beets, until a fork easily slides into the largest beet. Let cool for about 20 minutes, or until cool enough to handle.

3. Reduce the oven temperature to 150°C (300°F). Toast the hazelnuts in the oven for 12 to 15 minutes, or until the skins have darkened and are almost falling off. Place them on a damp dish-towel and rub vigorously until most of the skins fall off. Discard the skins and roughly chop the hazelnuts. Set aside.

4. Carefully unwrap the beets and trim the ends. Under cold running water, push the beet skins off with your fingers. Discard the skins.

5. Thinly slice the beets into 3mm rounds and arrange 7 to 12 beet slices on each of 3 plates.

6. Sprinkle a handful of toasted hazelnuts on top of each plate of beets. Add a drizzle of Balsamic Reduction and a drizzle of oil. Scatter the leaves from 1 to 2 sprigs thyme all over the beets on each plate, and serve.

Tip: To save some time, cook the beets the day before and refrigerate them until needed. When ready to use, slice the beets and serve cold or at room temperature.

long weekend grilled salad

FOR THE GRILLED VEGETABLES:
6 ears corn

Coconut oil or grapeseed oil, for brushing

Fine-grain sea salt and freshly ground black pepper

3 bell peppers (I use 1 red, 1 yellow, and 1 orange), quartered lengthwise

2 medium courgettes, halved lengthwise

FOR THE DRESSING:
3 tablespoons extra-virgin olive oil

3 tablespoons fresh lime juice

1 small clove garlic, minced

2 tablespoons minced fresh coriander leaves

1 teaspoon agave nectar or other liquid sweetener

¼ teaspoon fine-grain sea salt, plus more as needed

Freshly ground black pepper, to taste

TO ASSEMBLE:
1 avocado, halved and pitted

Fine-grain sea salt and freshly ground black pepper

Fresh coriander leaves, for serving (optional)

This salad is light, fresh, filling, and easy to throw together for any summer gathering. You can make it the day before – just throw it into a container and let the flavours marry overnight in the fridge. It travels well to any summer picnic or potluck gathering. Just give it a good shake or stir before serving so the dressing is evenly dispersed.

Serves 6

PREP TIME: 20 minutes • COOK TIME: 20 to 25 minutes
gluten-free, nut-free, soy-free, refined sugar-free, grain-free

1. Make the Grilled Vegetables: Brush each ear of corn with some coconut oil and season with salt and black pepper. Wrap each ear with foil, twisting the ends to secure.

2. Brush coconut oil on each piece of bell pepper and courgette and season with salt and black pepper.

3. Preheat a grill to medium for about 10 minutes. Place the corn, bell peppers, and courgettes on the grill, on the top rack, if possible. Grill for 10 to 15 minutes, rotating every 5 minutes. When the peppers and courgettes are lightly charred and tender, remove them from the grill and set aside on a platter. Continue grilling the corn for 10 to 15 minutes more, 20 to 25 minutes total. Set aside until cool enough to handle.

4. Make the Dressing: In a small bowl, whisk together the olive oil, lime juice, garlic, coriander, agave, salt, and black pepper to taste.

5. To assemble the salad, stand each ear of corn in a shallow dish and, using a chef's knife, remove the corn kernels from the cob by slicing downward along the length of the corn.

6. Chop the grilled bell peppers and courgettes and place them in a large bowl. Slice and add the avocado. Add the corn kernels and the dressing and toss to combine. Season generously with salt and black

pepper. (I usually end up adding another handful of chopped coriander, too, but that's optional.)

Tip: If you'd like to boost the protein content of this salad, feel free to add 1 425g can of black beans, drained and rinsed.

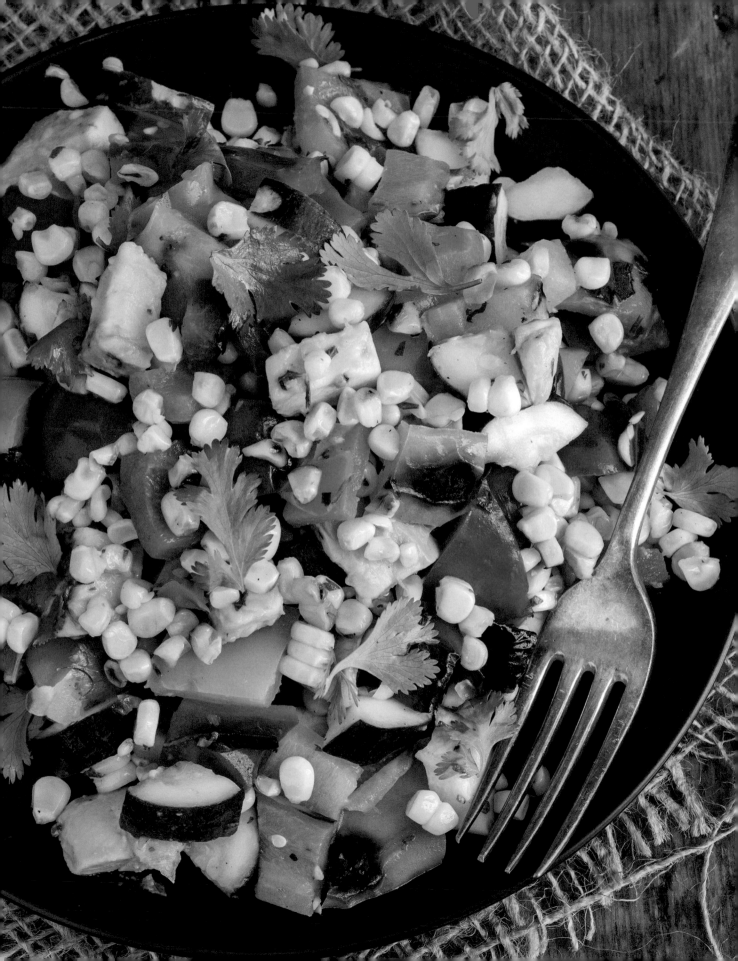

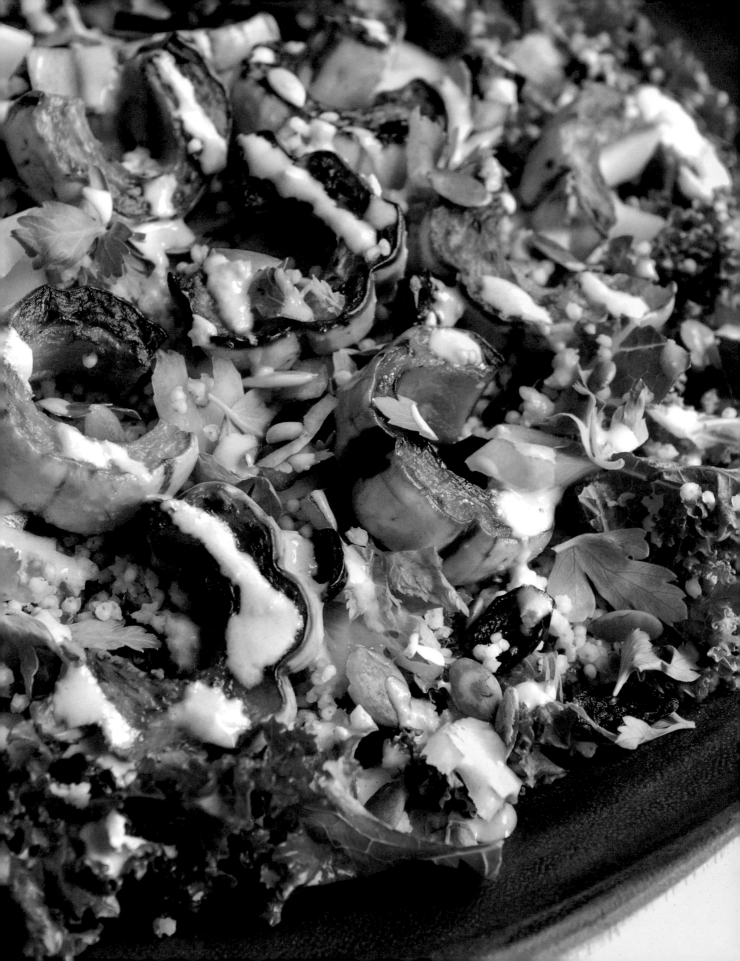

delicata squash, millet & kale salad with lemon-tahini dressing

2 delicata squash 790g to 900g total, halved lengthwise and seeded

1 tablespoon grapeseed or melted coconut oil

Fine-grain sea salt and freshly ground black pepper

200g uncooked millet or quinoa

½ to 1 bunch kale, stems removed, leaves torn into 2.5cm pieces

1 recipe Lemon-Tahini Dressing (see page 284)

75g diced red onions

75g chopped celery (about 1 large stalk)

10g fresh parsley leaves, roughly chopped

2 tablespoons dried cranberries

2 tablespoons raw or toasted pepita seeds

Delicata, or peanut, squash is my favourite squash to prepare because it has a thin, edible skin that doesn't require peeling, and it's easy to chop. In this cool-weather salad, kale and millet are topped with roasted delicata and a creamy lemon-tahini dressing. It's hearty and comforting while still being light and energizing. Don't despair if you can't find delicata squash; feel free to substitute your favourite squash in its place.

Serves 3

PREP TIME: 30 minutes • COOK TIME: 30 minutes
gluten-free, nut-free, soy-free, sugar-free

1. Preheat the oven to 220°C (425°F). Line a rimmed baking sheet with parchment paper.

2. Slice the squash crosswise into 2.5cm-wide pieces (they should be the shape of a U) and place them in a single layer on the prepared baking sheet. Drizzle them with the oil and toss to combine. Season generously with salt and pepper.

3. Roast the squash for about 30 minutes, flipping once halfway through the cooking time. The squash is ready when golden and fork-tender.

4. Meanwhile, cook the millet according to the instructions on page 302.

5. Place the kale in a large bowl and spoon 2 to 4 tablespoons of the Lemon-Tahini Dressing over the top. Massage the dressing into the kale with your hands until all the leaves are coated. Let the kale sit on the counter for at least 10 to 15 minutes (or longer, if desired) so the dressing can soften the kale leaves.

6. To assemble the salad, place the dressing-coated kale on a large serving plate. Spread the cooked millet over the top, followed by the onion, celery, parsley, roasted squash, cranberries, and pepita seeds. Drizzle with the rest of the dressing.

Tip: Try roasting the red onion along with the squash for a deep, caramelized flavour.

festive kale salad with sweet apple-cinnamon vinaigrette & pecan parmesan

FOR THE PECAN PARMESAN:
50g pecans, toasted

1½ teaspoons nutritional yeast

1½ to 3 teaspoons extra-virgin olive oil

¼ teaspoon fine-grain sea salt

FOR THE DRESSING:
3 tablespoons apple cider vinegar

2 tablespoons plus 1 teaspoon fresh lemon juice (from ½ lemon)

2 tablespoons pure maple syrup

½ teaspoon ground cinnamon

¼ teaspoon fine-grain sea salt

1 tablespoon extra-virgin olive oil or grapeseed oil

2 tablespoons unsweetened apple sauce

½ teaspoon minced fresh peeled ginger

TO ASSEMBLE:
1 bunch kale, destemmed and leaves torn into bite-size pieces

1 apple, cored and finely chopped

30g dried cranberries

80g pomegranate seeds (from about ½ pomegranate)

This salad, with its festive, cinnamon-maple dressing paired with fresh apple, dried cranberries, and pomegranate seeds, is perfect for the holidays. Kale is a sturdy green, so it travels well and won't wilt during transport. You can even make the salad the night before and leave it in the fridge to help soften the kale even more. I suggest adding the Pecan Parmesan just before you serve so it doesn't fall to the bottom of the salad.

Serves 4 to 6
PREP TIME: 20 to 25 minutes
COOK TIME: 7 to 9 minutes
gluten-free, soy-free, refined sugar-free, grain-free

1. Make the Pecan Parmesan: Preheat the oven to 150°C (300°F). Spread the pecans in a single layer on a rimmed baking sheet and toast in the oven for 7 to 9 minutes, until lightly golden and fragrant. Set aside to cool for 5 minutes.

2. In a mini food processor, combine the toasted pecans, nutritional yeast, oil, and salt and process until crumbly and combined. (You can also chop the pecans by hand and mix everything in a small bowl.) Set aside.

3. Make the Dressing: In a small bowl, whisk together the vinegar, lemon juice, maple syrup, cinnamon, salt, oil, apple sauce, and ginger until combined.

4. To assemble the salad, place the kale in a large salad bowl and pour on the dressing. With your hands, massage the dressing into the kale leaves until fully coated. Let stand for at least 30 minutes.

The kale will soften slightly during this time.

5. Top the kale with the apple, cranberries, and pomegranate seeds. Sprinkle the Pecan Parmesan over the salad just before serving.

❋

Tip: You can save the kale stems for juicing or smoothies, if you wish.

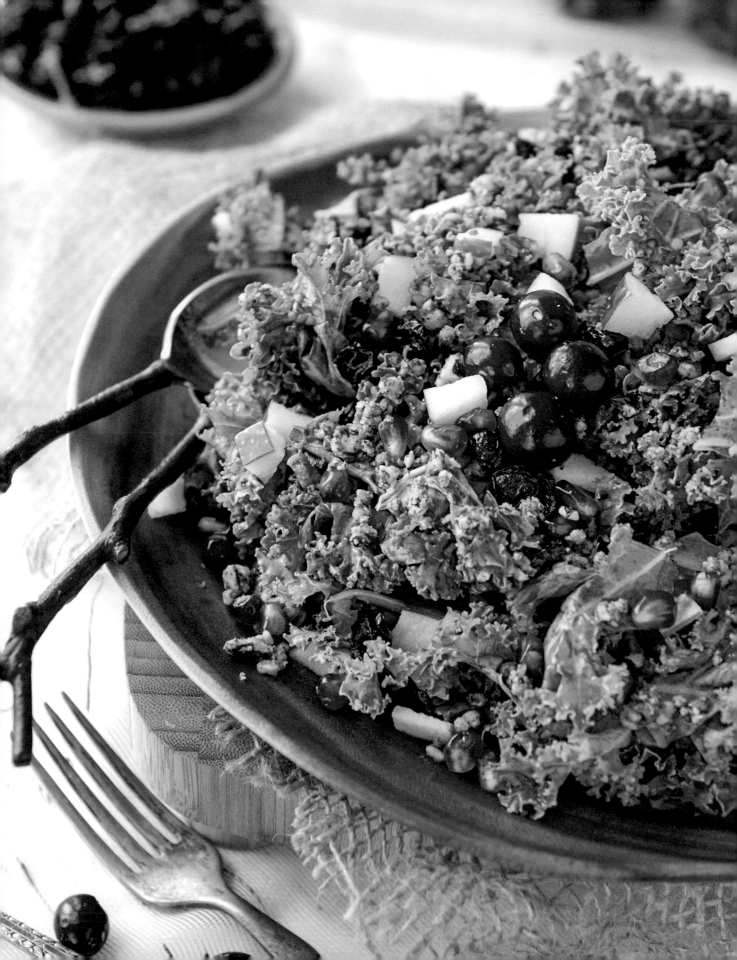

soup

I always say that making soup is easy, but nailing the perfect flavour combinations can be quite challenging. That's why I dedicate so much time to testing soup recipes. I want the flavours to really dazzle my palate, especially because I eat a lot of soup during the dreary cold winter months. These soup recipes will surely enliven your taste buds and soothe your soul when you need it the most! My Cream of Tomato Soup with Roasted Italian Chickpea Croutons (page 141) is one of my favourites. It reminds me of my favourite childhood soup, only it's much tastier and doesn't contain any animal products. Once you try my chickpea croutons, you may never see croutons the same way again!

Soups are a great way to nourish your health; I like to think of them as a multivitamin in a bowl. If you are looking for something to get your eating back on track, try the Eat Your Greens Detox Soup (page 139) or the fan-favourite On the Mend Spiced Red Lentil-Kale Soup (page 131). Both are great options to help you bounce back from a cold and feel your best, or you know, conquer the world.

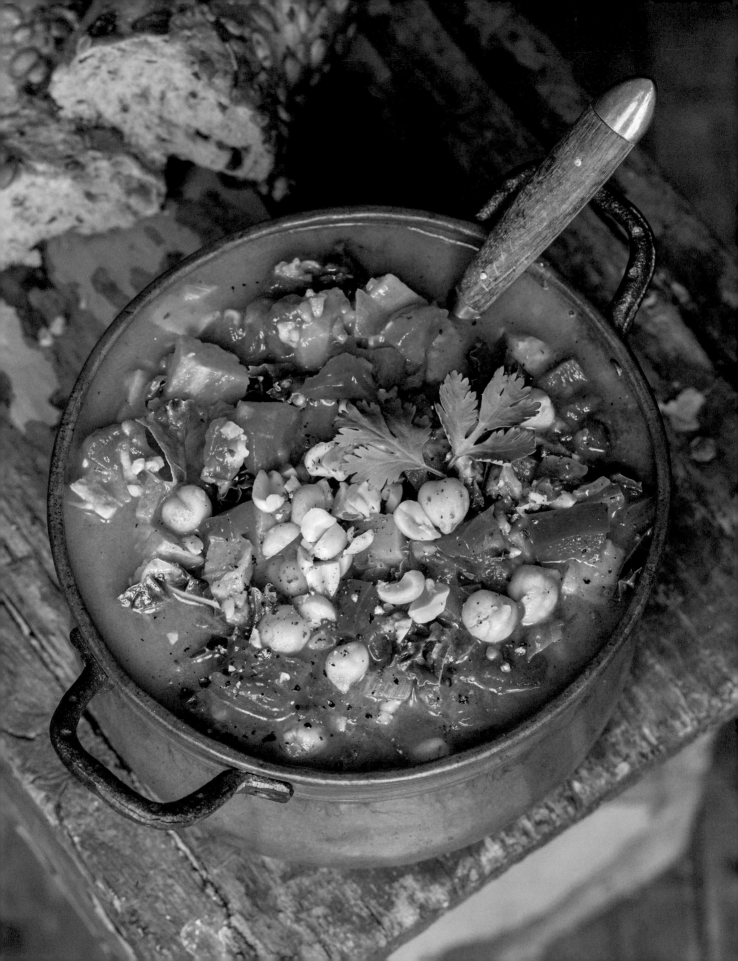

soul-soothing african peanut stew

1 teaspoon extra-virgin olive oil

1 medium sweet onion, diced

3 cloves garlic, minced

1 red bell pepper, diced

1 jalapeño, seeded, if desired, and diced (optional)

1 medium sweet potato, peeled and chopped into 1cm pieces

1 793g can diced tomatoes, with their juices

Fine-grain sea salt and freshly ground black pepper

85g natural peanut butter

1l vegetable broth, plus more as needed

1½ teaspoons chilli powder

¼ teaspoon cayenne pepper (optional)

1 425g can chickpeas, drained and rinsed

2 handfuls baby spinach or destemmed, torn kale leaves

Fresh coriander or parsley leaves, for serving

Roasted peanuts, for serving

Tip: Have some leftover cooked rice? This soup is fabulous with some stirred in.

Creamy, satisfying, and lightly spicy, you'll soon see why soul-soothing peanut butter and sweet potato are a match made in vegan heaven. If you are a fan of spicy food, I encourage you to add the optional cayenne pepper to give this recipe a bit more kick.

Serves 6

PREP TIME: 20 minutes • COOK TIME: 25 to 35 minutes

gluten-free, soy-free, sugar-free, grain-free

1. In a large saucepan, heat the oil over a medium heat. Add the onion and garlic and sauté for about 5 minutes, or until the onion is translucent.

2. Add the bell pepper, jalapeño (if using), sweet potato, and tomatoes with their juices. Raise the heat to medium-high and simmer for 5 minutes more. Season the vegetables with salt and black pepper.

3. In a medium bowl, whisk together the peanut butter and 250ml of the vegetable broth until no clumps remain. Stir the mixture into the vegetables along with the remaining 750ml broth, chilli powder, and the cayenne (if using).

4. Cover the pan with a lid and reduce the heat to medium-low. Simmer for 10 to 20 minutes, or until the sweet potato is fork-tender.

5. Stir in the chickpeas and spinach and cook until the spinach is wilted. Season with salt and black pepper to taste.

6. Ladle the stew into bowls and garnish with coriander or parsley and roasted peanuts.

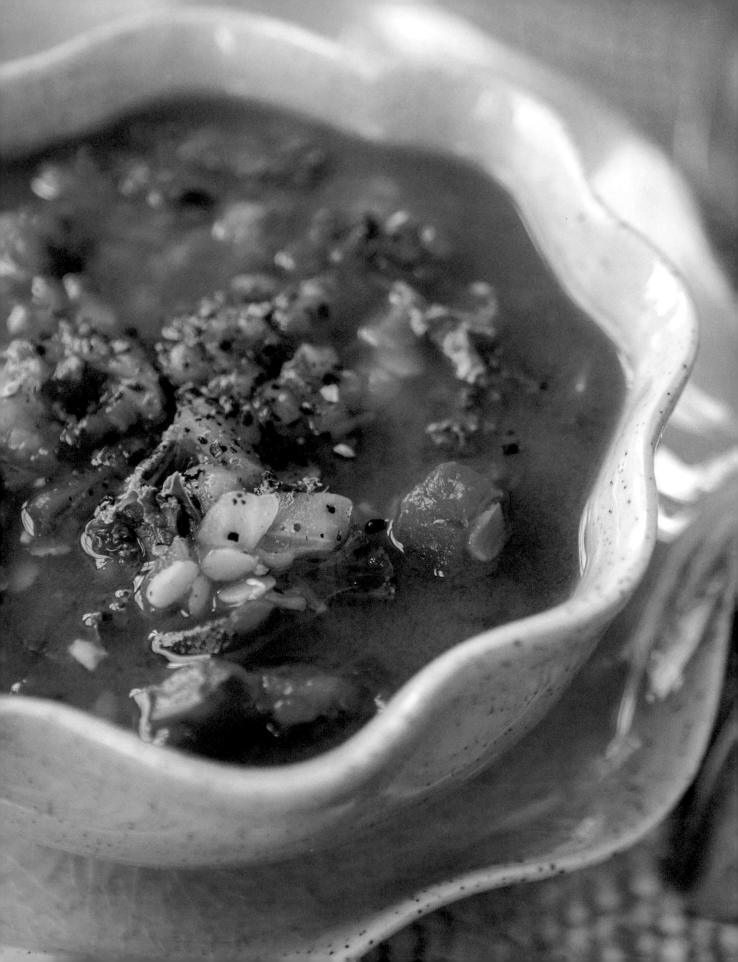

on the mend spiced red lentil-kale soup

1 teaspoon coconut oil or olive oil

1 sweet onion, diced

2 large cloves garlic, minced

3 stalks celery, diced

1 bay leaf

1¼ teaspoons ground cumin

2 teaspoons chilli powder

½ teaspoon ground coriander

¼ to ½ teaspoon smoked paprika, to taste

⅛ teaspoon cayenne pepper,
or to taste

1 396g can diced tomatoes, with their juices

1.25 to 1.5 litres vegetable broth, plus more as needed

190g uncooked red lentils, rinsed and drained

Fine-grain sea salt and freshly ground black pepper

2 handfuls destemmed torn kale leaves or spinach

Is it normal to want to guzzle broth? Well, it is now, my friends! Chilli powder, cumin, coriander, smoked paprika, and cayenne pepper create a downright irresistible and flavourful broth bursting with nutrition. It'll clear your nose in no time (but I wouldn't say it's overly spicy, unless, of course, you go crazy with the cayenne pepper). Since most vegetable soups don't hold me over very long, I added 190g of red lentils to this soup to ramp up the protein and fibre. Red lentils take a mere fifteen minutes to cook, and you can make everything in one pot, so it doesn't get much easier. Thanks to the lentils, this soup has more than 10 grams of protein per serving. Add some bread, crackers, or rice pilaf and you have yourself a nice little meal to enjoy with loved ones.

Serves 3

PREP TIME: 20 to 30 minutes • COOK TIME: 30 minutes
gluten-free, nut-free, soy-free, sugar-free, grain-free

1. In a large saucepan, heat the oil over a medium heat. Add the onion and garlic and sauté for 5 to 6 minutes, until the onion is translucent. Add the celery, season with salt, and sauté for a few minutes more.

2. Add the bay leaf, cumin, chilli powder, coriander, paprika, and cayenne and stir to combine. Sauté for a couple of minutes, until fragrant.

3. Stir in the tomatoes with their juices, the broth, and the lentils. Bring the mixture to the boil, then reduce the heat to medium and simmer, uncovered, for 20 to 25 minutes, until the lentils are tender and fluffy. Season with salt and pepper. Remove and discard the bay leaf.

4. Stir in the kale and cook for a few minutes more, until it has wilted. Serve immediately.

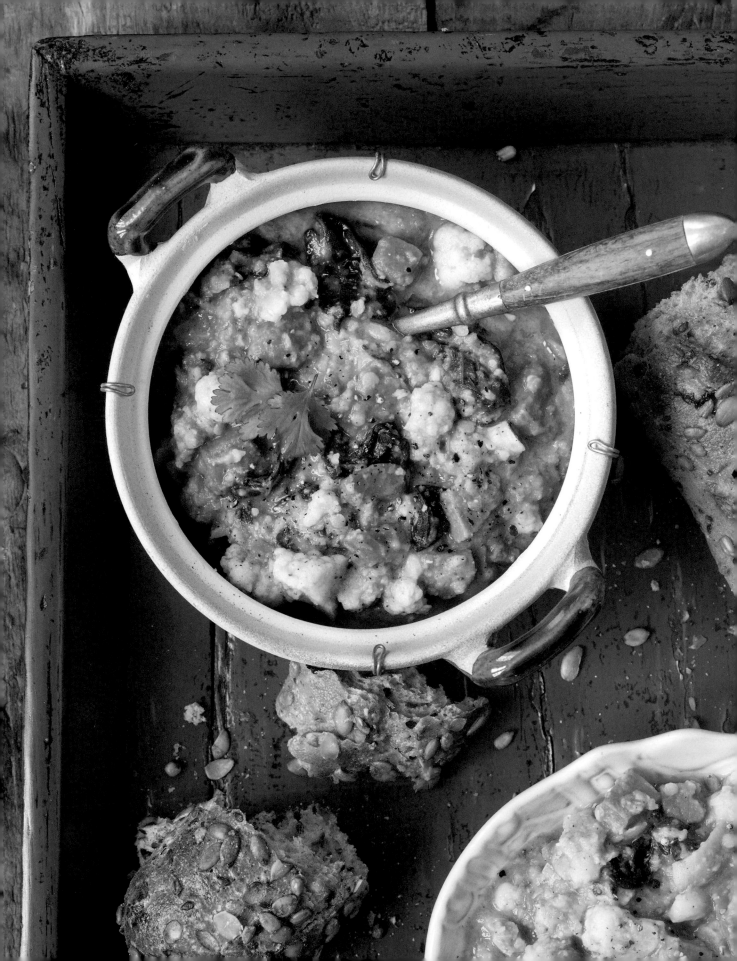

indian lentil-cauliflower soup

1 tablespoon coconut oil or
other oil

1 yellow onion, diced

2 large cloves garlic, minced

1 tablespoon minced peeled fresh ginger

1 to 2 tablespoons curry powder, to taste

1½ teaspoons ground coriander

1 teaspoon ground cumin

1.5 litres vegetable broth

190g uncooked red lentils, rinsed
and drained

1 medium cauliflower, chopped into
bite-size florets

1 medium sweet potato, peeled and diced

2 large handfuls baby spinach

¾ teaspoon fine-grain sea salt,
or to taste

Freshly ground black pepper

Chopped fresh coriander, for serving
(optional)

Why is it that the homeliest soups tend to taste the best? This soup isn't fancy-looking at first glance, but the flavour will make your taste buds bust out a dance routine. Or if you are like me, you might actually bust out a dance number mid-bite in the middle of the kitchen. (I never promised to be normal.) Ingredients like lentils and cauliflower make for a budget-friendly meal, while Indian spices like curry powder and fresh ginger are sure to warm you up on a cool day. The flavour gets better as it sits, so I tend to enjoy the leftovers even more.

Serves 4

PREP TIME: 30 minutes • COOK TIME: 32 to 37 minutes
gluten-free, nut-free, soy-free, sugar-free, grain-free

1. In a large saucepan, heat the oil over medium heat. Add the onion and garlic and sauté for 5 to 6 minutes, until translucent.

2. Stir in the ginger, 1 tablespoon of the curry powder, coriander, and cumin and sauté for 2 minutes more, until fragrant.

3. Add the broth and red lentils and stir to combine. Bring the mixture to a low boil, then reduce the heat and simmer for 5 minutes more.

4. Stir in the cauliflower and sweet potato. Cover and reduce the heat to medium-low. Simmer for 20 to 25 minutes, until the cauliflower and sweet potato are tender. Season with the salt and pepper, and add more curry powder, if desired. Stir in the spinach and cook until wilted.

5. Ladle the soup into bowls and top with coriander, if desired.

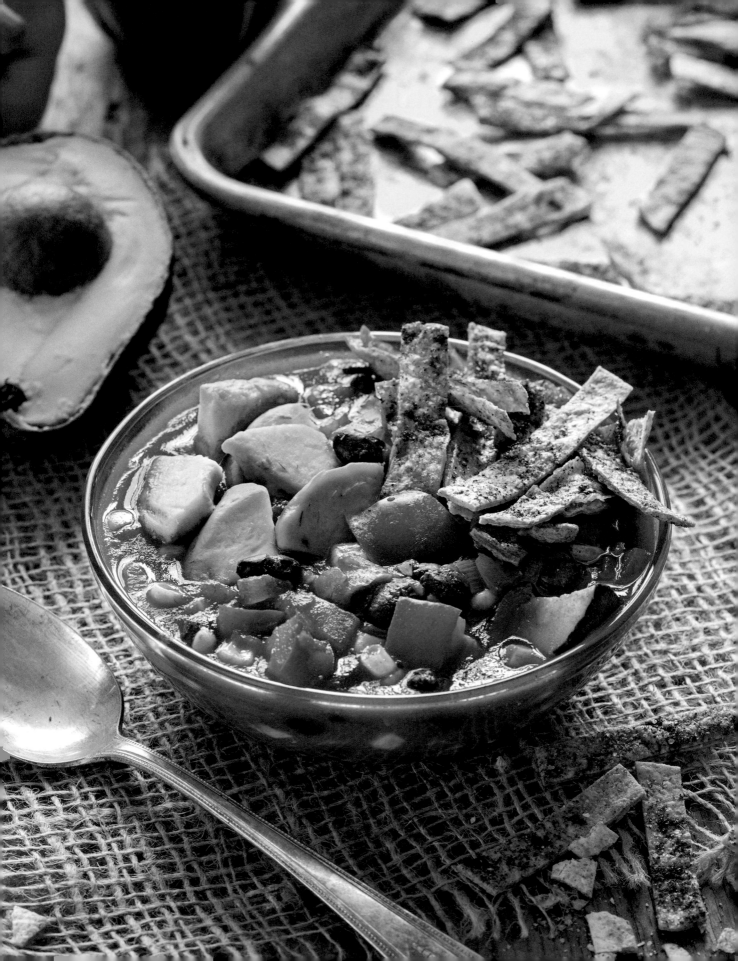

summer harvest tortilla soup

1 tablespoon extra-virgin olive oil

1 yellow onion, diced

3 large cloves garlic, minced

Freshly ground black pepper

1 large red bell pepper, diced

1 jalapeño, seeded, if desired, and diced (optional)

Kernels from 2 ears fresh corn, or 65g frozen corn kernels

1 medium courgette, chopped

1 680g jar or can crushed tomatoes

750ml vegetable broth

2 teaspoons ground cumin

½ teaspoon chilli powder

¼ teaspoon cayenne pepper

1 teaspoon fine-grain sea salt, or to taste

1 425g can black beans, drained and rinsed

OPTIONAL TOPPINGS:
Sliced avocado

Toasted tortilla strips (see Tips, below)

Fresh lime juice

Fresh coriander

This is a wonderful soup to help you make the transition from the end of summer into fall. It packs a bounty of summer produce like courgette, corn, peppers, and onions, so it's a great way to use up vegetables from the garden, a vegetable box subscription, or the farmer's market. I like to make a couple of batches of this soup at the end of the summer and freeze it for the cooler months.

Serves 4

PREP TIME: 20 minutes • COOK TIME: 25 to 30 minutes
gluten-free, nut-free, soy-free, sugar-free, grain-free option

1. In a large saucepan, heat the oil over a medium heat. Add the onion and garlic and sauté for about 5 minutes. Season with salt and black pepper.

2. Stir in the bell pepper, jalapeño (if using), corn kernels, and courgette. Raise the heat to medium-high and sauté for 10 minutes more.

3. Add the crushed tomatoes, broth, cumin, chilli powder, and cayenne and stir well. Season with salt and black pepper.

4. Bring the soup to a low boil and reduce the heat to medium. Simmer, uncovered, for 10 to 15 minutes, until the vegetables are tender. Stir in the black beans and simmer for 2 minutes more.

5. Ladle the soup into bowls and garnish.

Tips: To make toasted tortilla strips, follow the recipe for Spiced Toasted Pitta Chips on page 91, but use tortillas instead of pitta bread and slice the tortillas into thin 5cm strips before toasting. For a heartier soup, try adding brown or wild rice.

If you are avoiding canned tomato products, look for crushed tomatoes in a jar. Eden Organics is a great organic brand.

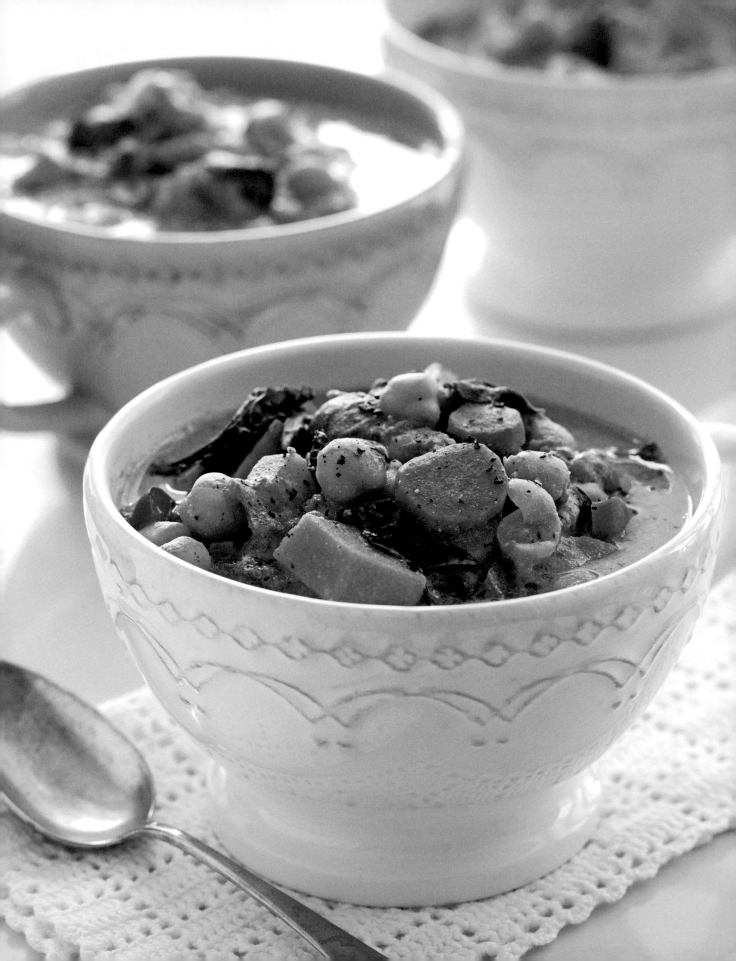

10-spice vegetable soup with cashew cream

120g raw cashews, soaked (see page 11)

1.5 litres vegetable broth

2 teaspoons extra-virgin olive oil

4 cloves garlic, minced

1 sweet or yellow onion, diced

3 medium carrots, chopped

1 red bell pepper, chopped

225g peeled and chopped sweet potato, regular potato, or butternut squash

2 stalks celery, chopped

1 793g can diced tomatoes, with their juices

1 tablespoon 10-Spice Blend (see page 284)

Fine-grain sea salt and freshly ground black pepper, to taste

2 bay leaves

30g to 60g baby spinach or destemmed torn kale leaves (optional)

1 425g can chickpeas or other beans, drained and rinsed (optional)

This is quite possibly the ultimate bowl of comfort food, made with a decadent, creamy broth and loaded with an array of health-boosting spices. It's really hard to stop at one bowl! Be sure to soak the raw cashews in water the night before (or for at least three to four hours) so they are ready when you plan to make the soup.

Serves 6

PREP TIME: 30 minutes • COOK TIME: 30 minutes

gluten-free, soy-free, sugar-free, grain-free

1. In a blender, combine the soaked and drained cashews with 250ml of the vegetable broth and blend on the highest speed until smooth. Set aside.

2. In a large saucepan, heat the oil over a medium heat. Add the garlic and onion and sauté for 3 to 5 minutes, or until the onion is translucent.

3. Add the carrots, bell pepper, potato, celery, diced tomatoes with their juices, remaining 1.25 litres of broth, the cashew cream, and the 10-Spice Blend. Stir well to combine. Bring the mixture to the boil and then reduce the heat to medium-low. Season with salt and black pepper and add the bay leaves.

4. Simmer the soup, uncovered, for at least 20 minutes, until the vegetables are tender. Season with salt and black pepper. During the last 5 minutes of cooking, stir in the spinach and beans, if desired. Remove and discard the bay leaves before serving.

Tip: If you don't have the ingredients on hand to make the 10-Spice Blend, feel free to use your favorite store-bought Cajun or Creole seasoning mix and add to taste.

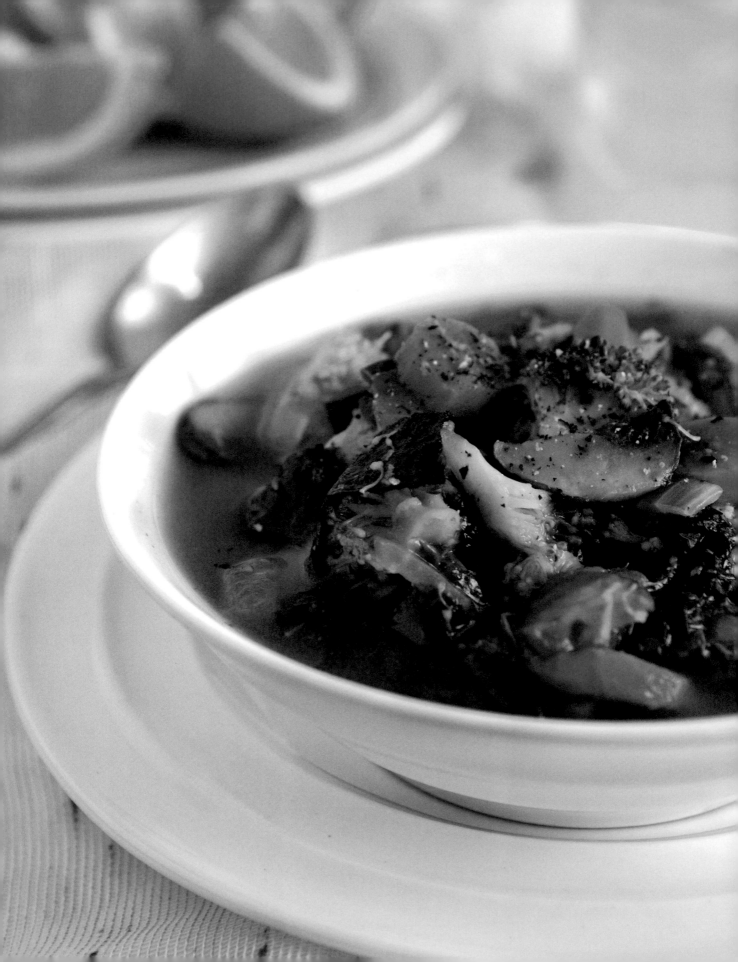

eat your greens detox soup

1½ teaspoons coconut oil or olive oil

1 sweet onion, diced

3 cloves garlic, minced

225g sliced cremini or white button mushrooms

150g chopped carrots

250g chopped broccoli florets

Fine-grain sea salt and freshly ground black pepper, to taste

1½ to 3 teaspoons grated peeled fresh ginger

½ teaspoon ground turmeric

2 teaspoons ground cumin

⅛ teaspoon ground cinnamon

1.25 litres vegetable broth

2 large nori seaweed sheets, cut into 2.5cm strips (optional)

70g torn kale leaves

Fresh lemon juice, for serving (optional)

Calling all vegetable lovers! This soup is great if you want to cleanse and detoxify your body, especially before or after an indulgent holiday. It's packed with detoxifying and immunity-boosting ingredients like broccoli, ginger, mushrooms, kale, nori, and garlic, and will get your healthy eating right back on track.

Serves 3

PREP TIME: 25 minutes • COOK TIME: 20 to 30 minutes
gluten-free, nut-free, soy-free, sugar-free, grain-free

1. In a large saucepan, heat the oil over a medium heat. Add the onion and garlic and sauté for about 5 minutes, until the onion is soft and translucent.

2. Add the mushrooms, carrots, and broccoli and stir to combine. Season generously with salt and pepper and sauté for 5 minutes more.

3. Stir in the ginger, turmeric, cumin, and cinnamon and sauté for 1 to 2 minutes, until fragrant.

4. Add the broth and stir to combine. Bring the mixture to a boil and then reduce the heat to medium-low and simmer until the vegetables are tender, 10 to 20 minutes.

5. Just before serving, stir in the nori (if using) and kale and cook until wilted. Season with salt and pepper and a squeeze of fresh lemon juice, if desired.

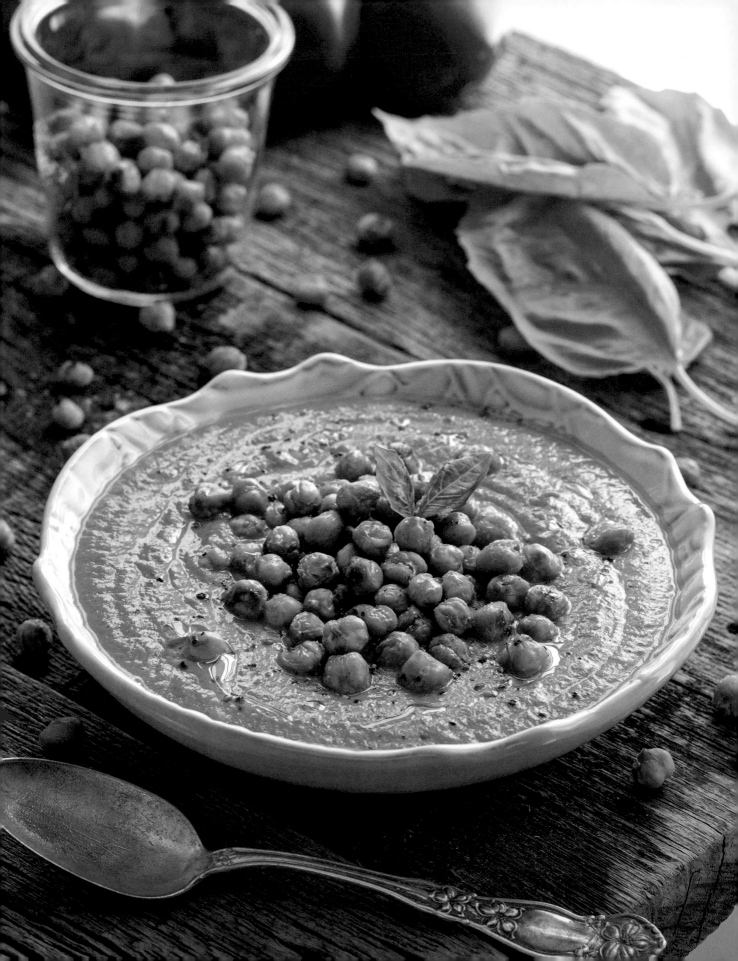

cream of tomato soup with roasted italian chickpea croutons

FOR THE CHICKPEA CROUTONS:
1 425g can chickpeas, drained and rinsed

1 teaspoon grapeseed oil or melted coconut oil

½ teaspoon dried oregano

⅛ teaspoon cayenne pepper

1 teaspoon garlic powder

¼ teaspoon onion powder

¾ teaspoon fine-grain sea salt or Herbamare

FOR THE TOMATO SOUP:
1 tablespoon extra-virgin olive oil

1 small to medium yellow onion, diced

2 large cloves garlic, minced

75g raw cashews, soaked (see page 11)

500ml vegetable broth

1 793g can whole peeled tomatoes, with their juices

15g oil-packed sun-dried tomatoes, drained

3 to 4 tablespoons tomato paste

½ to 1 teaspoon dried oregano

¾ to 1 teaspoon fine-grain sea salt

½ teaspoon freshly ground black pepper, plus more as needed

¼ to ½ teaspoon dried thyme

FOR SERVING:
Fresh basil leaves

Olive oil

Freshly ground black pepper

This is a classic cream-based tomato soup, revamped to be good for you and free of animal products. Blending a small amount of soaked cashews into the soup transforms the tomato base into a luxurious, creamy soup, and the sun-dried tomatoes add depth of flavour to the tomato base. And with the crunchy Italian chickpea 'croutons,' there are no traditional bread croutons required. Be sure to soak the raw cashews in water the night before (or for at least three to four hours) so they are ready when you plan to make the soup.

Makes 2 litres
PREP TIME: 20 minutes
COOK TIME: 30 to 40 minutes
gluten-free, soy-free, sugar-free, grain-free

1. Make the Chickpea Croutons: Preheat the oven to 220°C (425°F). Line a large rimmed baking sheet with paper towels. Place the chickpeas on the paper towels and place a couple of paper towels on top. Roll them around until any liquid on them has been absorbed. Discard the paper towels.

2. Transfer the chickpeas to a large bowl and stir in the grapeseed oil, oregano, cayenne, garlic powder, onion powder, and salt. Line the baking sheet with parchment paper and then spread the chickpeas in an even layer on the baking sheet.

3. Bake for 15 minutes. Give the pan a shake from side to side and cook for 15 to 20 minutes more, watching closely, until the chickpeas are lightly charred and golden.

4. Let cool on the baking sheet for at least 5 minutes. The chickpeas will crisp up as they cool.

5. Make the Tomato Soup: In a large saucepan, heat the olive oil over a medium heat. Add the onion and garlic and sauté for 5 to 6 minutes, or until the onion is translucent.

6. In a blender, combine the soaked cashews and the broth and blend on high speed until creamy and smooth. Add the garlic-onion mixture, tomatoes and their juices, sun-dried tomatoes, and tomato paste and blend on high until smooth.

7. Pour the tomato mixture into the saucepan in which you cooked the onions and set the pan over medium-high heat. Bring the mixture to a simmer, then stir in the oregano, salt, pepper, and thyme, all to taste.

8. Gently simmer over a medium heat, uncovered, for 20 to 30 minutes, until the flavours have developed.

9. Ladle the soup into bowls and top each with the Chickpea Croutons. Garnish with minced fresh basil leaves, a drizzle of olive oil, and freshly ground black pepper.

Tips: The chickpeas will lose their crispness in the soup, so be sure to add them just before you sit down to eat – or you can even add the chickpeas as you eat the soup.

If you have leftover chickpeas, make sure they're cool, then pop them into a baggie or container and throw them in the freezer. Freezing the chickpeas seems to retain their crispness better than leaving them at room temperature. To reheat, simply pop the frozen chickpeas into the oven at 220°C (425°F) for 5 minutes or so, until thawed. Voilà – instant roasted chickpeas!

....
oh she glows

mains

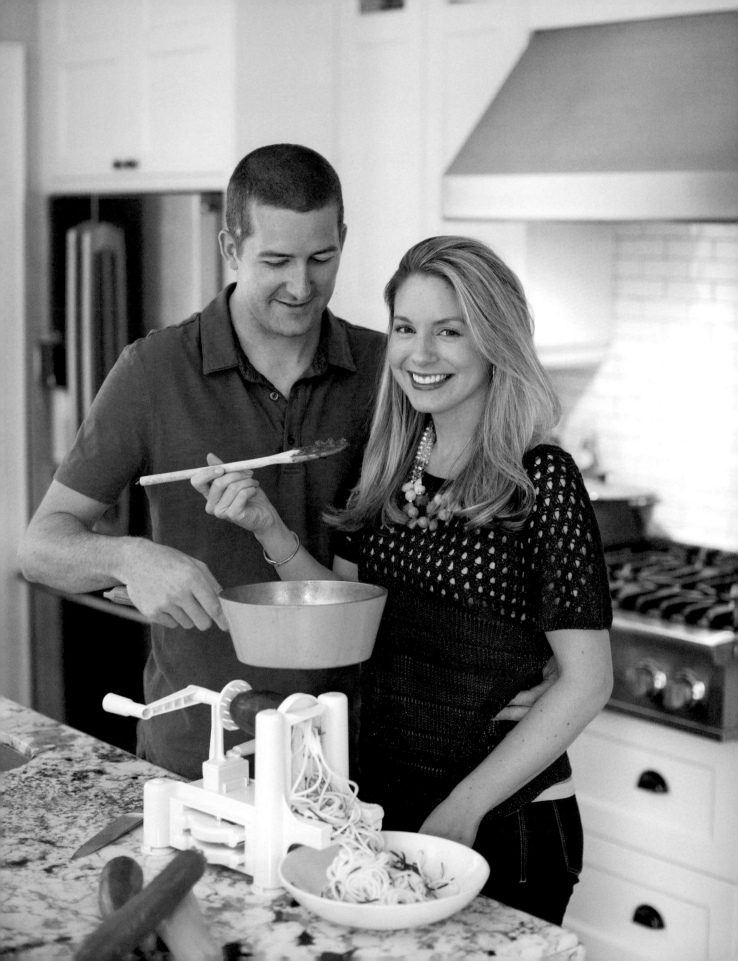

When I develop recipes, I feel it's important that they please meat-eaters and vegans alike; if they don't, they don't make the cut or I work diligently until they pass the test. I cook for many omnivores, so I'm confident that the meals in this chapter are ones that virtually anyone can enjoy. We can all agree on one thing: We like food that tastes good! You'll find a mixture of healthy weeknight meals such as Immunity-Boosting Tomato Sauce with Mushrooms (page 161), 15-Minute Creamy Avocado Pasta (page 173), and Quick & Easy Chana Masala (page 163), as well as more elaborate dishes like the popular Lentil-Walnut Loaf (page 167) and Crowd-Pleasing Tex-Mex Casserole (page 149). If you are looking for a burger to win over a crowd, Our Favourite Veggie Burger (page 155) does just that, or for a quicker option, the Grilled Portobello Burger (page 169) is mouthwatering as well.

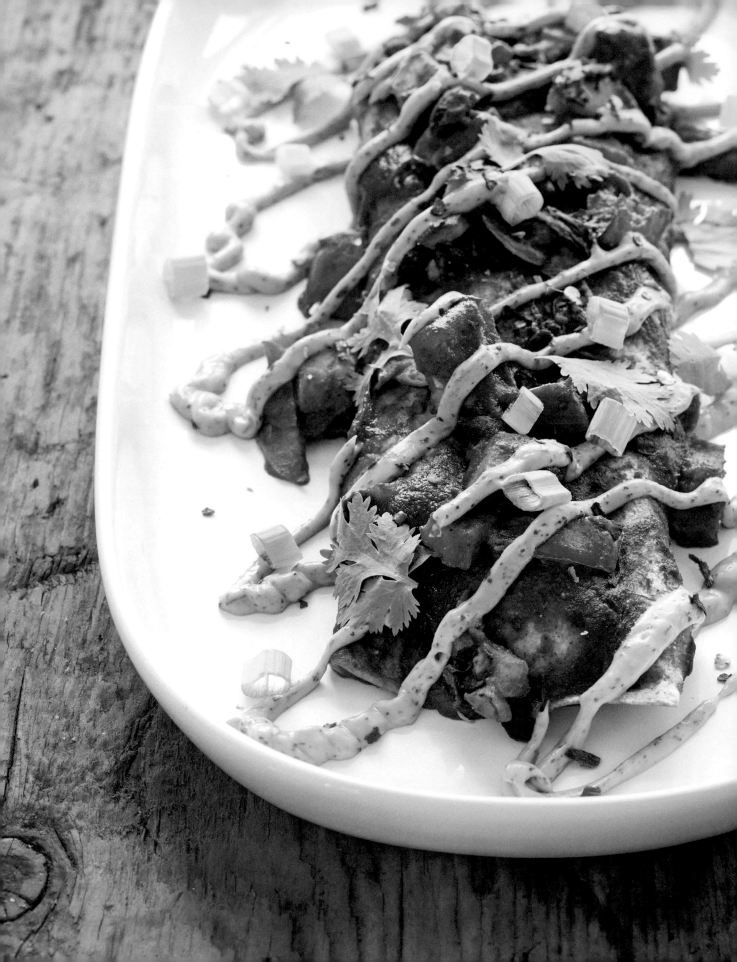

sweet potato & black bean enchiladas with avocado-coriander cream sauce

FOR THE ENCHILADAS:

300g sweet potato, peeled and chopped small

1 tablespoon extra-virgin olive oil

1 red onion, chopped

2 large cloves garlic, minced

Fine-grain sea salt and freshly ground black pepper

1 bell pepper, chopped

1 425g can black beans, drained and rinsed

2 large handfuls spinach, roughly chopped

625ml 5-Minute Enchilada Sauce (see page 300) or store-bought

1 tablespoon fresh lime juice

1 teaspoon chilli powder, or to taste

½ teaspoon ground cumin

½ teaspoon kosher salt, or to taste

5 sprouted-grain tortilla wraps or gluten-free corn tortillas

FOR THE AVOCADO-CORIANDER CREAM SAUCE:

25g fresh coriander

1 medium avocado, pitted

2 tablespoons lime juice

¼ teaspoon fine-grain sea salt

½ teaspoon garlic powder

Fresh coriander leaves, for serving

Sliced green onion, for serving

You just might forget all about cheese when you take your first bite of these sweet potato, black bean, and spinach enchiladas. Creamy avocado sauce flavoured with coriander, lime, garlic, and cumin takes this dish over the top, smothering the enchiladas in a decadent, but healthy, creamy topping. No cheese required. And the 5-Minute Enchilada Sauce is so flavourful and easy to make, you may never use store-bought sauce again!

Serves 5

PREP TIME: 30 minutes   •   COOK TIME: 20 to 25 minutes
gluten-free option, nut-free, soy-free, sugar-free

1. Preheat the oven to 180°C (350°F). Lightly grease a large 2.8-litre rectangular baking dish.

2. Make the Enchiladas: Place the sweet potato in a medium saucepan and add enough water to cover. Bring the water to a boil, then reduce the heat to medium-high and simmer for 5 to 7 minutes, or until fork-tender. Drain and set aside.

3. In a large frying pan, heat the oil over a medium heat. Add the onion and garlic and sauté for about 5 minutes, until the onion is translucent. Season with sea salt and black pepper.

4. Add the bell pepper, cooked sweet potato, black beans, and spinach. Raise the heat to medium-high and cook for a few minutes more, or until the spinach is wilted.

5. Remove the pan from the heat and stir in 60ml of the enchilada sauce, the lime juice, chilli powder, cumin, and kosher salt.

6. Spread 250ml of the enchilada sauce evenly over the bottom of the prepared baking dish. Scoop 245g of the sweet potato filling onto each tortilla. Roll up the tortillas and place them seam side down in the baking dish. Spread the remaining enchilada sauce over the tortillas. If you have leftover filling, spoon it on top of the tortillas as well.

7. Bake the enchiladas, uncovered, for 20 to 25 minutes, until the sauce is a deep red colour and the enchiladas are heated through.

8. Meanwhile, make the Avocado-Coriander Cream Sauce: In a food processor, process the coriander until minced. Add the avocado, lime juice, sea salt, garlic powder, and 3 tablespoons of water and process until creamy, stopping to scrape down the bowl as needed.

9. When the enchiladas are ready to serve, plate them individually and drizzle or spread some of the Avocado-Coriander Cream Sauce on top of each. Garnish with coriander and green onion, if desired.

crowd-pleasing tex-mex casserole

FOR THE TEX-MEX SPICE BLEND:

1 tablespoon chilli powder

1½ teaspoons ground cumin

1 teaspoon smoked sweet paprika, or
½ teaspoon regular paprika

¼ teaspoon cayenne pepper, plus more as
needed

1¼ teaspoons fine-grain sea salt

¼ teaspoon ground coriander (optional)

FOR THE CASSEROLE:

1½ teaspoons extra-virgin olive oil

1 red onion, diced

3 cloves garlic, minced

1 orange bell pepper, diced

1 red bell pepper, diced

1 jalapeño, seeded, if desired, and diced

Fine-grain sea salt and freshly ground
black pepper

90g fresh or frozen corn

1 396g can diced tomatoes, with their
juices

250ml tomato sauce or tomato puree

120 to 200g chopped kale leaves or baby
spinach

1 425g can black beans, drained and
rinsed

500g cooked wild rice blend or brown rice
(see page 302)

50g vegan shredded cheese, such as Daiya

1 to 2 handfuls corn tortilla chips, crushed

OPTIONAL TOPPINGS:
Sliced green onions • Salsa • Avocado •
Corn chips • Cashew Cream
(see page 281)

Out of all the casseroles I tested for this book, this is the dish that won everyone over – men and children included. Similar to a burrito in a bowl, this casserole is the perfect mix of flavour and comfort. It never ceases to amaze me how a meal with a few simple ingredients like rice, beans, and vegetables can turn out so incredible. While the casserole is good on its own, I find it's even better with a generous amount of toppings like sliced avocado, salsa, corn chips, green onion, and Cashew Cream (see page 281), so go wild.

Serves 6
PREP TIME: 30 minutes
COOK TIME: 20 minutes (plus rice cooking time)
gluten-free, nut-free, soy-free, sugar-free

1. Make the Tex-Mex Spice Blend: In a small bowl, combine the chilli powder, cumin, paprika, cayenne, salt, and coriander (if using). Set aside.

2. Make the Casserole: Preheat the oven to 190°C (375°F). Oil a large 5-litre casserole dish.

3. In a large wok, heat the oil over a medium heat. Add the onion, garlic, bell peppers, and jalapeño and sauté for 7 to 8 minutes, until softened. Season with salt and black pepper.

4. Stir in the Tex-Mex Spice Blend, corn, diced tomatoes and their juices, tomato sauce, kale, beans, rice, and 25g of the vegan shredded cheese. Sauté for a few minutes and season with more salt and black pepper, if desired.

5. Pour the mixture into the prepared casserole dish and smooth out the top. Sprinkle the crushed chips over the casserole mixture along with the remaining cheese. Cover with a lid or foil and bake for 15 minutes.

6. Uncover the casserole dish and cook for 5 to 10 minutes more, until bubbly and lightly golden around the edges.

7. Scoop the casserole into bowls and add your desired toppings.

Tip: I suggest cooking the rice ahead of time to make this recipe come together much faster. You can even use precooked frozen rice (just thaw it before using).

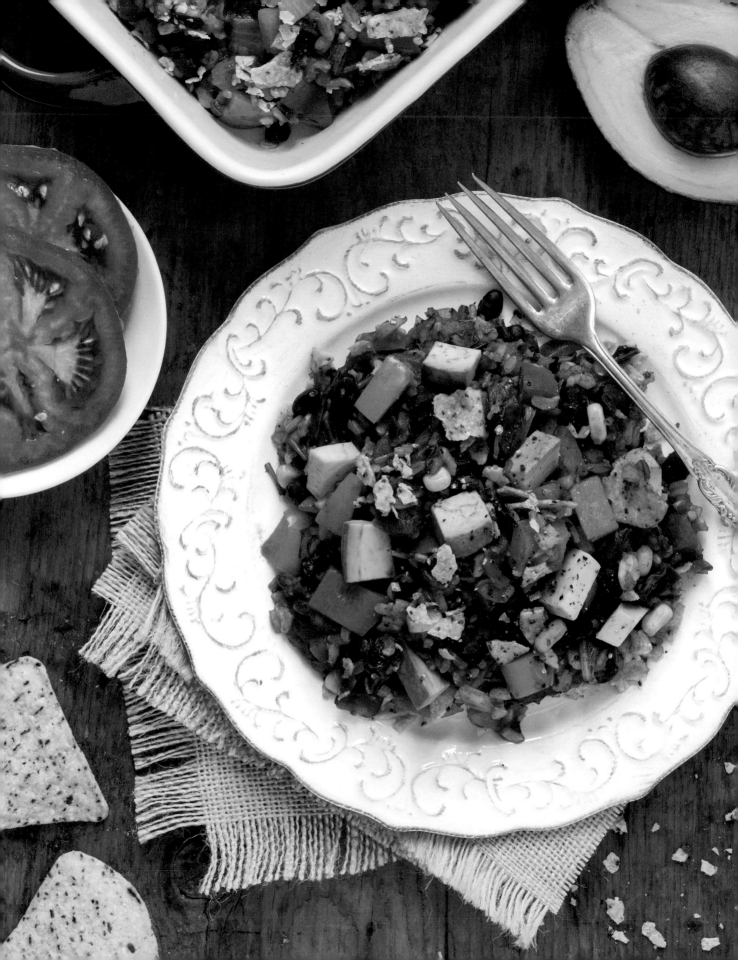

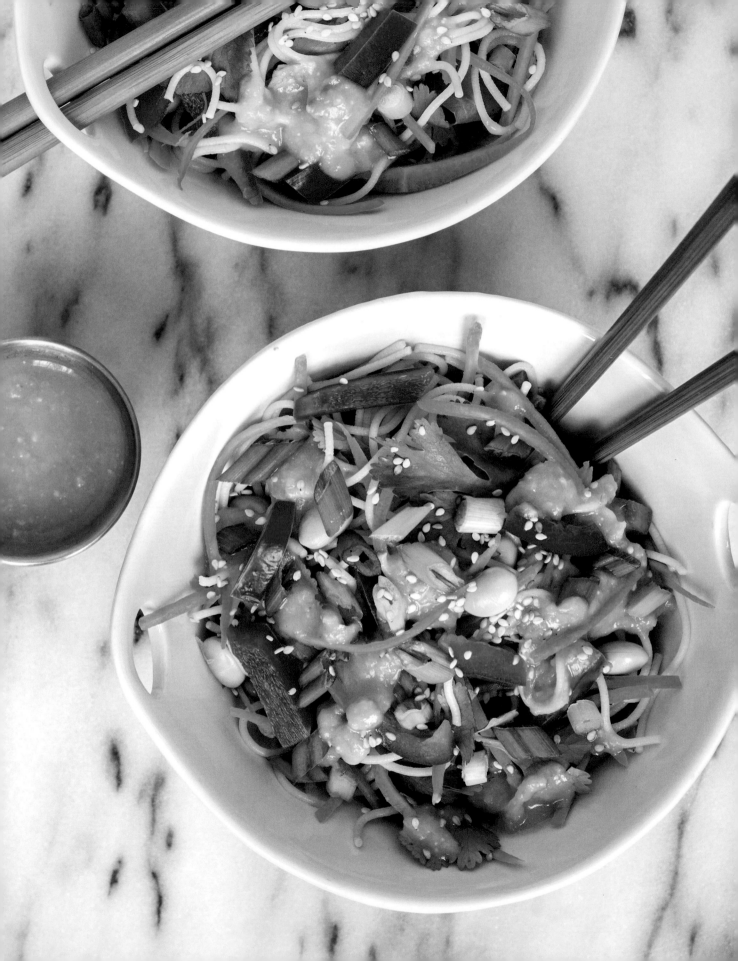

empowered noodle bowl, two ways: thai peanut & orange-maple miso

FOR THE THAI PEANUT SAUCE:

1 large clove garlic

2 tablespoons toasted sesame oil

3 tablespoons natural smooth peanut butter or almond butter

2 teaspoons grated fresh ginger (optional)

3 tablespoons fresh lime juice, plus more as needed

2 tablespoons plus 1 teaspoon low-sodium tamari

1 to 2 teaspoons granulated sugar

FOR THE ORANGE-MAPLE MISO DRESSING:

3 tablespoons light miso

2 tablespoons rice vinegar

1 tablespoon toasted sesame oil

1 tablespoon tahini

60ml fresh orange juice

1 tablespoon water

1 teaspoon maple syrup

FOR THE SALAD:

115g gluten-free soba (buckwheat) noodles

Extra-virgin olive oil, for the noodles

1 454g bag frozen shelled edamame, thawed

1 red bell pepper, diced

½ seedless (English) cucumber, diced

1 carrot, julienned

4 green onions, chopped, plus more for serving

10g fresh coriander leaves, chopped

Sesame seeds, for serving

Choosing between my Thai Peanut and Orange-Maple Miso sauces felt like choosing a favourite child, so of course I had to include both of them in the book. It's always fun to have options, don't you think? The miso dressing is a great choice if you're looking for a nut-free noodle dressing, and the Thai peanut dressing is perfect if you are a big fan of creamy peanut butter or almond butter.

Serves 4

PREP TIME: 25 minutes • COOK TIME: 5 to 9 minutes

gluten-free, nut-free option (Orange-Maple Miso Dressing), soy-free option

1. Make the Thai Peanut Sauce: In a mini or regular food processor, combine the garlic, sesame oil, peanut butter, ginger (if using), lime juice, tamari, sugar (if using), and 2 to 3 tablespoons of water. Process until combined.

OR

Make the Orange-Maple Miso Dressing: In a mini or regular food processor, combine the miso, vinegar, sesame oil, tahini, orange juice, water, and maple syrup and process until well combined.

2. Make the Salad: Cook the soba noodles according to the instructions on the package. Be sure not to overcook them – they should only take 5 to 9 minutes, depending on the brand. Drain the noodles and rinse them under cold water. Transfer the noodles to a large bowl and toss them with a drizzle of extra-virgin olive oil (this prevents the noodles from sticking together).

3. Add the edamame, bell pepper, cucumber, carrot, green onions, and coriander to the bowl with the noodles and toss until well combined.

4. Pour your desired amount of the dressing over the salad and toss to coat. (Any leftover dressing will keep in an airtight container in the refrigerator for up to 1 week.)

5. Portion the salad into 4 bowls and garnish each serving with a sprinkle of sesame seeds and some green onions. Serve any leftover dressing on the side.

Tips: For a soy-free Thai Peanut Sauce, replace the tamari with coconut aminos. To make this dish completely soy-free, omit the edamame as well.

If you need a soy-free and gluten-free miso, look for chickpea miso. My go-to brand is South River Miso and it's absolutely lovely in this sauce.

For a raw version, serve this noodle bowl with spiralized or julienned courgette (see page 23), instead of the soba noodles.

our favorite veggie burger

3 tablespoons ground flaxseed

1 425g can black beans, drained and rinsed

150g grated carrots or sweet potato

10g finely chopped fresh parsley or coriander leaves

2 large cloves garlic, minced

60g finely chopped red or yellow onions

75g sunflower seeds, toasted, if preferred

75g gluten-free rolled oats, processed into a flour

25g spelt breadcrumbs or Sprouted-Grain Breadcrumbs (see page 279), optional

½ tablespoon extra-virgin olive oil

1 to 2 tablespoons tamari or coconut aminos, to taste

1 teaspoon chilli powder

1 teaspoon dried oregano

1 teaspoon ground cumin

¾ to 1 teaspoon fine-grain sea salt

Freshly ground black pepper

These sturdy and flavourful veggie burgers have all the elements my family and I love in a veggie burger – they're chewy and hearty, and they hold together when cooking. Veggie burgers are fantastic because they keep well for the entire week and can be frozen after cooking for quick and easy meals down the road. Serve them with toasted multiseed buns, with lettuce wraps, or crumbled over salads. Really, you can't go wrong no matter which way you serve them. This recipe is inspired by Shelley Adams, author of the Whitewater Cooks cookbook series. You can find Shelley online at whitewatercooks.com – thanks, Shelley!

Serves 8

PREP TIME: 25 minutes

COOK TIME: 30 to 35 minutes

nut-free, sugar-free, gluten-free option, soy-free option

1. Preheat the oven to 180°C (350°F). Line a baking sheet with parchment paper.

2. In a small bowl, combine the flaxseed with 75ml warm water and set aside for 5 to 10 minutes, until thickened.

3. In a large bowl, mash the black beans into a paste, leaving a few beans intact for texture. Stir in the rest of the ingredients and the flaxseed mixture. Adjust the seasonings to taste, if desired. Mix well until combined.

4. With slightly wet hands, shape the dough into 8 patties. Pack the dough tightly to help it hold together during cooking and place the patties on the prepared baking sheet.

5. Bake the patties for 15 minutes, gently flip them, and bake for 15 to 20 minutes more, until the patties are firm and golden. Alternatively, grill the veggie burgers: Preheat a grill over a medium

heat. Prebake the patties in the oven for about 15 minutes at 180°C (350°F), then place them on the grill. Grill on each side for a few minutes until lightly golden.

6. Serve with toasted buns or lettuce leaf 'wraps.'

Tips: To make these burgers gluten-free, use certified gluten-free oats, gluten-free tamari, and omit the breadcrumbs.

To make these burgers soy-free, use a soy-free tamari (such as a brown rice-based tamari) or coconut aminos.

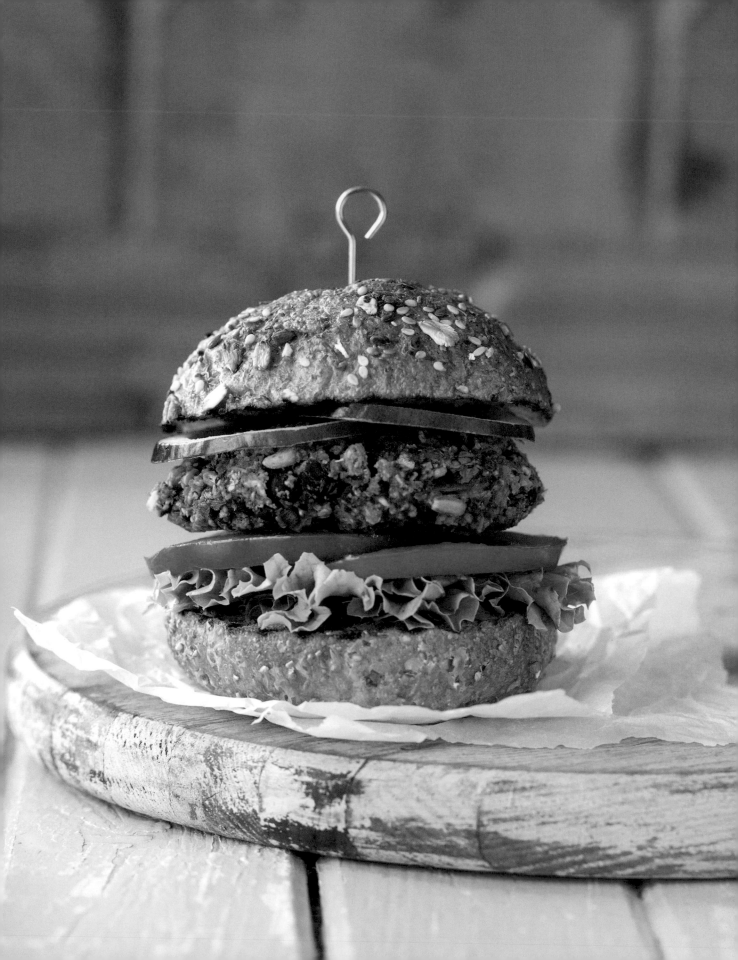

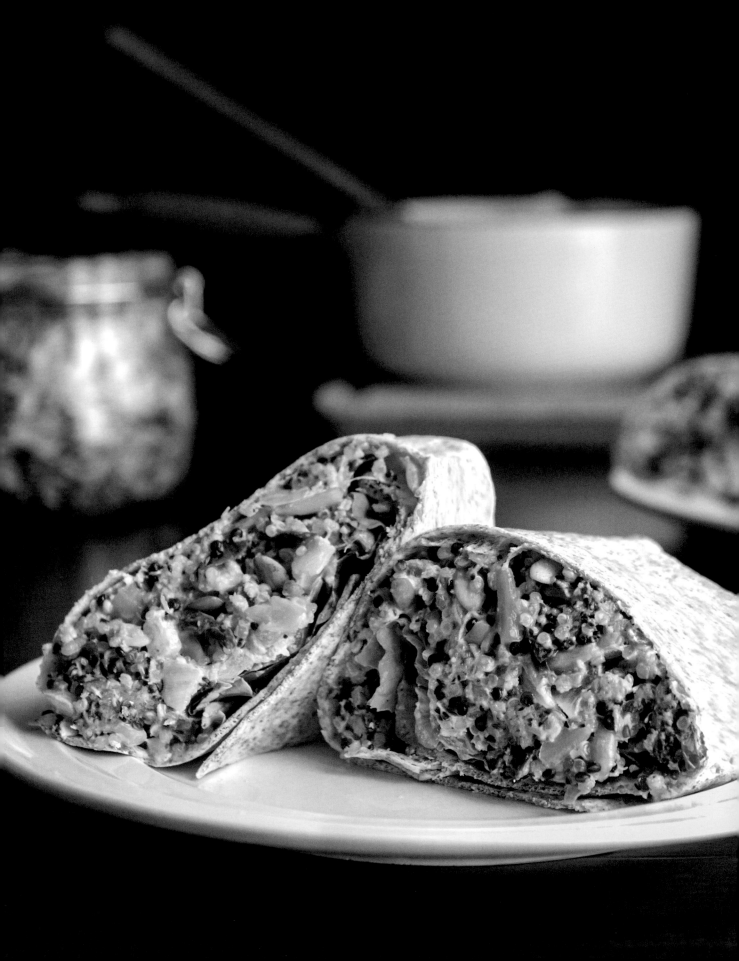

broccoli & cashew cheese-quinoa burrito

FOR THE CASHEW CHEESE SAUCE:
125g raw cashews

1 clove garlic

125ml unsweetened, unflavoured almond milk

30g nutritional yeast

1½ teaspoons Dijon mustard

1 teaspoon white wine vinegar or lemon juice

¼ teaspoon onion powder

½ teaspoon fine-grain sea salt

FOR THE BURRITO:
170g uncooked quinoa

1 teaspoon extra-virgin olive oil

1 clove garlic, minced

225g diced sweet onions

Fine-grain sea salt and freshly ground black pepper

75g diced celery

350g diced broccoli florets

3 to 4 tablespoons chopped, oil-packed sun-dried tomatoes, to taste

¼ teaspoon red pepper flakes (optional)

4 soft gluten-free tortillas or large lettuce leaves

This burrito reminds me of a broccoli and cheese casserole, only it's combined with protein-packed gluten-free quinoa instead of pasta and my velvety dairy-free cheese sauce. Stuff this cheesy, warm filling into a wrap for the ultimate comfort-food burrito.

Serves 4

PREP TIME: 25 minutes • COOK TIME: 20 to 30 minutes

gluten-free, soy-free, sugar-free

1. Make the Cashew Cheese Sauce: Place the cashews in a bowl and add enough water to cover. Soak the cashews for at least 3 to 4 hours, preferably longer if you have time. Drain and rinse the cashews.

2. In a food processor or blender, combine the soaked cashews, garlic, almond milk, nutritional yeast, mustard, vinegar, onion powder, and salt and process until smooth. The sauce should be very thick.

3. Make the Burrito: Cook the quinoa according to the instructions on page 302. Set aside.

4. In a large wok, heat the oil over a medium heat. Add the garlic and onion and sauté for about 5 minutes, until the onion is translucent. Season with salt and pepper.

5. Stir in the celery, broccoli, and sun-dried tomatoes, to taste. Sauté over a medium-high heat until the broccoli is tender, 10 to 15 minutes.

6. Add the cooked quinoa and cheese sauce and stir to combine with the vegetables. Add red pepper flakes, if desired. Cook until heated through, 5 to 10 minutes. Spoon the mixture onto the tortillas, wrap, and serve. You can also grill or press the burrito before serving, if desired.

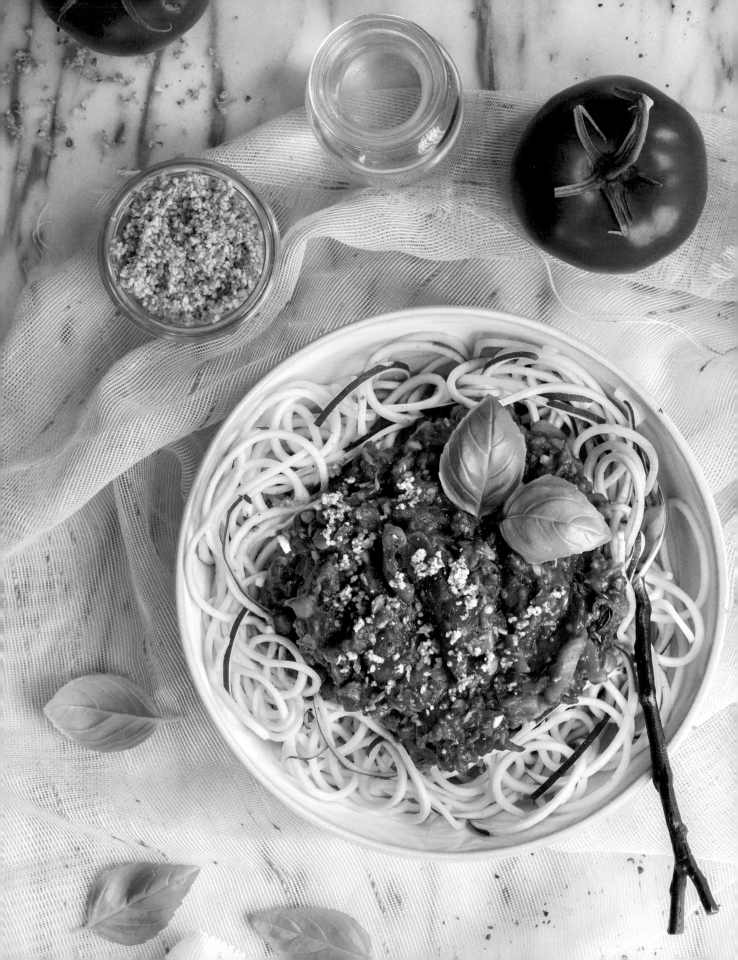

immunity-boosting tomato sauce with mushrooms

1 tablespoon extra-virgin olive oil

1 sweet onion, diced

4 cloves garlic, minced

225g sliced cremini mushrooms

10g packed fresh basil, chopped

1 793g can whole or diced tomatoes, with their juices

6 to 8 tablespoons tomato paste

½ to 1 teaspoon fine-grain sea salt, to taste

1½ teaspoons dried oregano

½ teaspoon dried thyme

¼ teaspoon red pepper flakes or cayenne pepper (optional)

2 tablespoons chia seeds (optional)

200g cooked lentils (optional)

This is my go-to spaghetti sauce recipe, the one I rely on for topping pasta, courgette noodles, and spaghetti squash. The mushrooms are optional, but they provide a hearty, meaty texture as well as anti-inflammatory and immune system–boosting nutrients. I like to stir in a couple of tablespoons of chia seeds to help thicken the sauce and boost the healthy omega-3 fatty acids. This is easily one of the healthiest and heartiest sauces to come out of my kitchen!

Makes 1.25 to 1.5 litres

PREP TIME: 20 minutes • COOK TIME: 30 minutes

gluten-free, nut-free, soy-free, sugar-free, grain-free

1. In a large saucepan, heat the oil over a medium heat. Add the onion and garlic and stir to combine. Sauté for 5 to 6 minutes, until the onion is translucent. Season with salt and pepper.

2. Stir in the mushrooms and raise the heat to medium-high. Cook for 5 to 10 minutes, until much of the liquid released by the mushrooms has cooked off.

3. Add the basil, whole peeled tomatoes and their juices, tomato paste, salt, oregano, and thyme. Stir to combine. With a wooden spoon, break up the whole tomatoes into chunks, bigger or smaller depending on how chunky you like your sauce. Skip this process if using diced tomatoes. Add the red pepper flakes, the chia seeds, and lentils, if desired, and stir to combine.

4. Reduce the heat to medium. Simmer the sauce, stirring every so often, for 15 to 20 minutes.

5. Serve over pasta and enjoy!

Tip: I like to add 200g of cooked lentils (or crumbled tofu or tempeh) into this sauce to boost the protein content. If you have kids and they don't like the texture of lentils, give the lentils a few whirls in the food processor before adding them to the sauce. They will have a texture very similar to ground beef and also work wonderfully for thickening the sauce.

....
oh she glows

quick & easy chana masala

1 tablespoon coconut oil or olive oil

1½ teaspoons cumin seeds

1 yellow onion, diced

1 tablespoon minced fresh garlic

1 tablespoon minced peeled fresh ginger

1 green serrano chilli pepper, seeded, if preferred, and minced

1½ teaspoons garam masala

1½ teaspoons ground coriander

½ teaspoon ground turmeric

¾ teaspoon fine-grain sea salt, plus more as needed

¼ teaspoon cayenne pepper (optional)

1 793g can whole peeled or diced tomatoes, with their juices

1 793g can chickpeas, or 492g cooked chickpeas (see page 290), drained and rinsed

195g dry/uncooked basmati rice, for serving (see page 302 for cooking instructions)

Fresh lemon juice, for serving

Fresh coriander, chopped, for serving

I'm a huge fan of chana masala, a spicy Indian chickpea dish, but I always thought that it would be too time-consuming to make at home due to the long list of spices the recipe requires. Once I purchased a few spices to add to my collection, there was no excuse not to make this easy, budget-friendly dish, and as it turns out, throwing them into a frying pan really isn't very time-consuming after all! You'll be wondering why you didn't make it sooner. To streamline this recipe, be sure to prep all the ingredients before starting; the cooking process for this dish moves quickly and it helps to have everything ready to go.

Serves 4

PREP TIME: 15 to 20 minutes

COOK TIME: 20 minutes

gluten-free, nut-free, soy-free, sugar-free, grain-free option

1. In a large wok or saucepan, heat the oil over a medium heat. When a drop of water sizzles upon hitting the pan, reduce the heat to medium-low and add the cumin seeds. Stir and toast the seeds for a minute or two until golden and fragrant, watching carefully to avoid burning.

2. Raise the heat to medium and stir in the onion, garlic, ginger, and serrano chilli. Cook for a few minutes or so, then stir in the garam masala, coriander, turmeric, salt, and cayenne (if using), and cook for 2 minutes more.

3. Add the whole peeled tomatoes and their juices and break them apart with a wooden spoon (skip if using diced tomatoes). You can leave some chunks of tomato for texture.

4. Raise the heat to medium-high and add the chickpeas. Bring the mixture to a simmer and cook for 10 minutes or longer to allow the flavours to develop.

5. Serve over cooked basmati rice, if desired, and garnish with a squeeze of fresh lemon juice and some chopped coriander just before serving.

Tips: To thicken the tomato gravy, place a ladle of the curry in a mini processor and process until almost smooth. Stir this back into the curry to thicken.

For a grain-free option, serve the chana masala atop a baked potato.

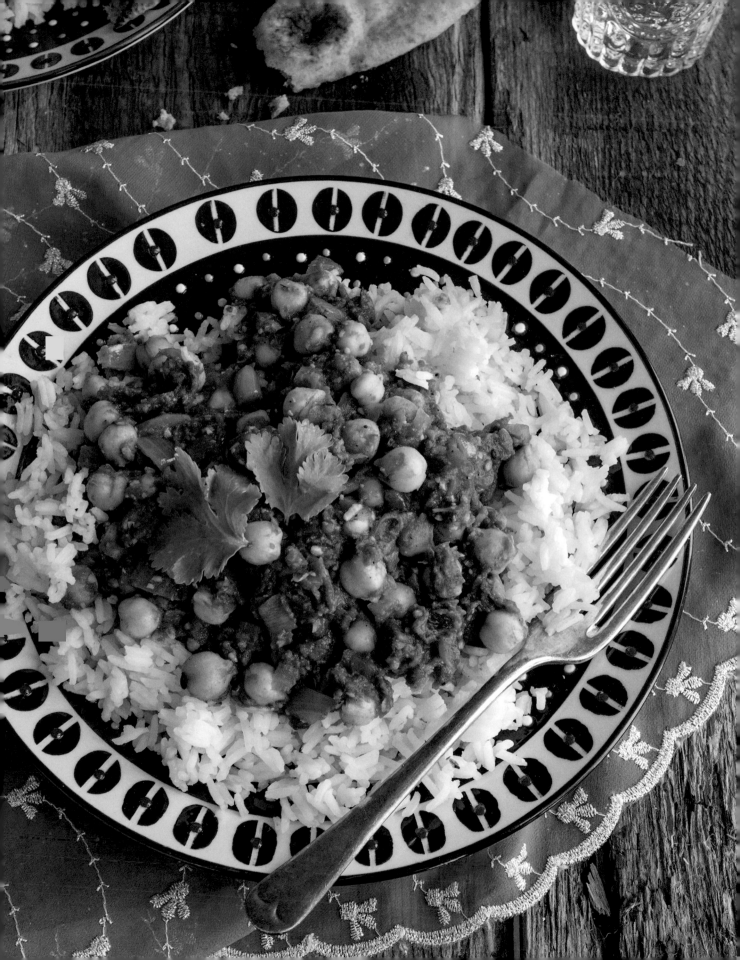

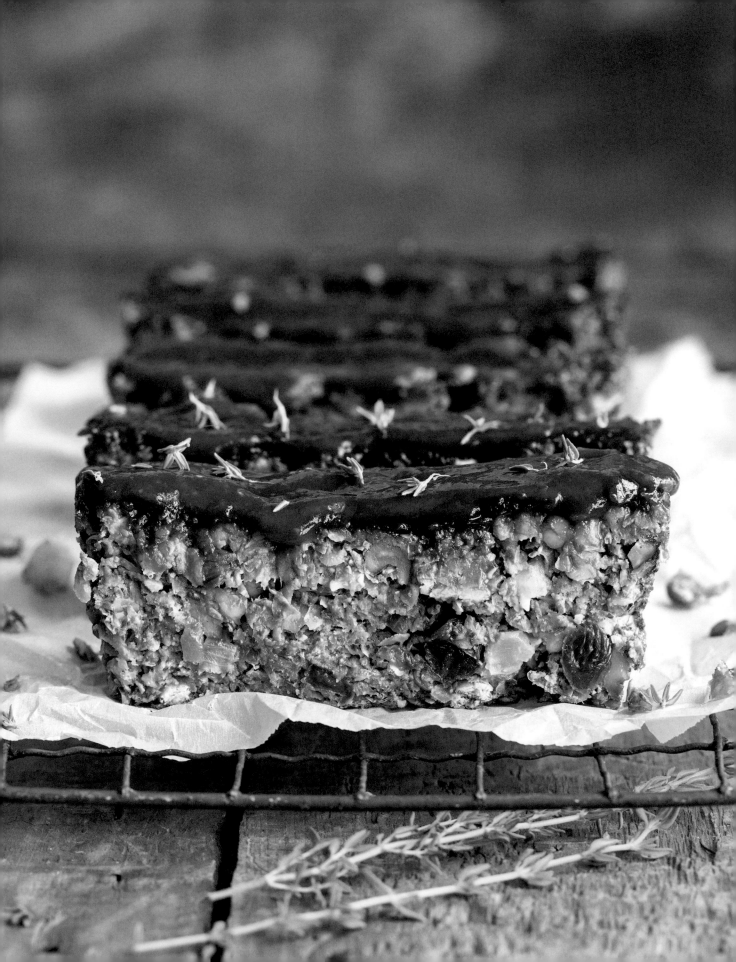

lentil-walnut loaf

FOR THE LOAF:

210g uncooked green lentils

125g shelled walnuts halves, finely chopped

3 tablespoons ground flaxseed

1 teaspoon extra-virgin olive oil

3 cloves garlic, minced

1 medium yellow onion, finely chopped

Fine-grain sea salt for seasoning, plus 1 teaspoon sea salt, or to taste

Freshly ground black pepper, for seasoning, plus ¼ teaspoon freshly ground black pepper

100g finely chopped celery

150g grated carrot

40g grated peeled sweet apple (optional)

60g raisins

50g gluten-free oat flour

45g spelt breadcrumbs or Sprouted-Grain Breadcrumbs (page 279)

1 teaspoon dried thyme, or 2 teaspoons fresh thyme leaves

1 teaspoon dried oregano

¼ teaspoon red pepper flakes (optional)

FOR THE BALSAMIC-APPLE GLAZE:

60ml ketchup

2 tablespoons unsweetened apple sauce or apple butter

2 tablespoons balsamic vinegar

1 tablespoon pure maple syrup

Fresh thyme leaves, for garnish (optional)

This Lentil-Walnut Loaf is adapted from a recipe by Terry Walters – multitalented cookbook author, motivational speaker, and food educator. Raved about by blog readers, husbands, children, and recipe testers alike, this recipe has inspired many people to claim the result is better than traditional meat loaf. Of course I agree! It's a bit of a fussy recipe, but it's always worth the time and effort. Be sure to finely chop all the vegetables so the loaf holds together well. I love to serve it with Cauliflower Mashed Potatoes (see page 207), apple sauce, and/or steamed greens. Thank you, Terry, for the inspiration!

Serves 8

PREP TIME: 40 to 45 minutes

COOK TIME: 55 to 60 minutes

soy-free, refined sugar-free, gluten-free option

1. Make the Loaf: Cook the lentils according to the instructions on page 302. In a food processor, process the cooked lentils for a few seconds into a coarse paste, leaving some lentils intact for texture. Set aside.

2. Preheat the oven to 160°C (325°F). Spread the walnuts on a rimmed baking sheet and toast them in the oven for 9 to 11 minutes. Set the walnuts aside, and raise the oven temperature to 180°C (350°F). Line a 22 x 12cm loaf tin with parchment paper.

3. In a large wok, heat the oil over medium heat. Add the garlic and onion and sauté for about 5 minutes, or until the onions are translucent. Season with salt and black pepper. Add the celery, carrot, apple (if using), and raisins. Sauté for about 5 minutes more.

4. Carefully stir in the processed lentils, flaxseed, walnuts, oat flour, breadcrumbs, thyme, oregano, 1 teaspoon salt, ¼ teaspoon black pepper, and red pepper flakes, if using. Stir until well combined and adjust the seasoning to taste, if desired.

5. Press the lentil mixture firmly and evenly into the prepared loaf tin. Use a pastry roller to roll it out smooth and compact the mixture.

6. Make the Balsamic-Apple Glaze: In a small bowl, whisk together the ketchup, apple sauce, balsamic vinegar, and maple syrup until combined. Spread the glaze over the loaf with a spoon or pastry brush.

7. Bake, uncovered, for 50 to 60 minutes, until the edges are lightly browned. Cool the loaf in the pan for 10 minutes. Slide a butter knife around the edge of the loaf and gently lift it out of the pan (using the parchment paper) and onto a cooling rack. Cool for 30 minutes more before slicing. If the loaf is sliced while warm, it may crumble slightly, but it holds together well when fully cooled. Garnish with fresh thyme leaves before serving, if desired.

Tip: For a gluten-free loaf, use gluten-free breadcrumbs instead of spelt breadcrumbs.

grilled portobello burger with sun-dried tomato kale-hemp pesto

FOR THE PORTOBELLO CAPS:

2 medium portobello mushrooms

2 tablespoons balsamic vinegar

2 tablespoons plus 1½ teaspoons fresh lemon juice

2 tablespoons extra-virgin olive oil

1 clove garlic, minced

1 teaspoon dried oregano

1 teaspoon dried basil

¼ teaspoon fine-grain sea salt

¼ teaspoon freshly ground black pepper

FOR THE SUN-DRIED TOMATO KALE-HEMP PESTO:

1 clove garlic

70g lightly packed destemmed kale leaves

10g oil-packed sun-dried tomatoes

15g hemp seeds

1 tablespoon fresh lemon juice

1 tablespoon olive oil

¼ teaspoon fine-grain sea salt

OPTIONAL TOPPINGS:

Caramelized onions (see Tips, page 170)

Avocado slices

Kale or lettuce leaves

Sliced tomatoes

The ultimate summertime burger! If you are a fan of juicy portobello mushroom caps, you will go crazy over this simple, but memorable, burger recipe. The tangy balsamic vinegar and lemon herb marinade enhance the mushrooms, and you pair them with a savoury sun-dried tomato kale-hemp pesto and succulent caramelized onions. Oh, mama mia. Serve it in a toasted bun or slice it and wrap in a couple of lettuce leaves.

Serves 2, with leftover pesto

PREP TIME: 15 to 20 minutes plus 1 hour marinating

COOK TIME: 10 minutes

gluten-free, nut-free, soy-free, sugar-free, grain-free

1. Remove the stems from the mushrooms by twisting the stem until it pops off. Discard the stem or save it for another use, such as a stir-fry. With a small spoon, scrape out and discard the black gills. Rub the cap with a damp dishcloth to remove any debris. In a large bowl, whisk together the vinegar, lemon juice, oil, garlic, oregano, basil, salt, and pepper. Add the portobello caps and toss to coat them in the marinade. Marinate the mushrooms for 30 to 60 minutes, tossing them every 15 minutes. (You can also marinate them overnight, if desired.)

2. Meanwhile, make the Sun-dried Tomato Kale-Hemp Pesto: In a food processor, pulse the garlic until minced. Add the kale leaves, sun-dried tomatoes, hemp seeds, lemon juice, olive oil, salt, and 2 tablespoons of water and process until smooth, stopping and scraping down the sides of the bowl as necessary.

3. Preheat a grill pan or an outdoor grill over a medium-high heat. Grill the portobello caps for 4 to 5 minutes per side, until lightly charred and tender.

4. Serve the portobello caps on a toasted bun or sliced up in a lettuce wrap topped with a generous amount of the pesto, and additional toppings of your choice. Any leftover pesto will keep in an airtight container in the refrigerator for at least 1 week. It's great on sandwiches, wraps, pasta, and more!

Tips: To make caramelized onions, thinly slice a sweet or yellow onion and sauté it over a medium heat in 1 tablespoon of oil until golden and lightly browned, but not burned. It usually takes about 30 minutes to bring out the onion's natural sugars.

For a grain-free option, serve the portobello bunless or slice caps and serve in lettuce wraps.

Use a gluten-free bun to make this recipe gluten-free.

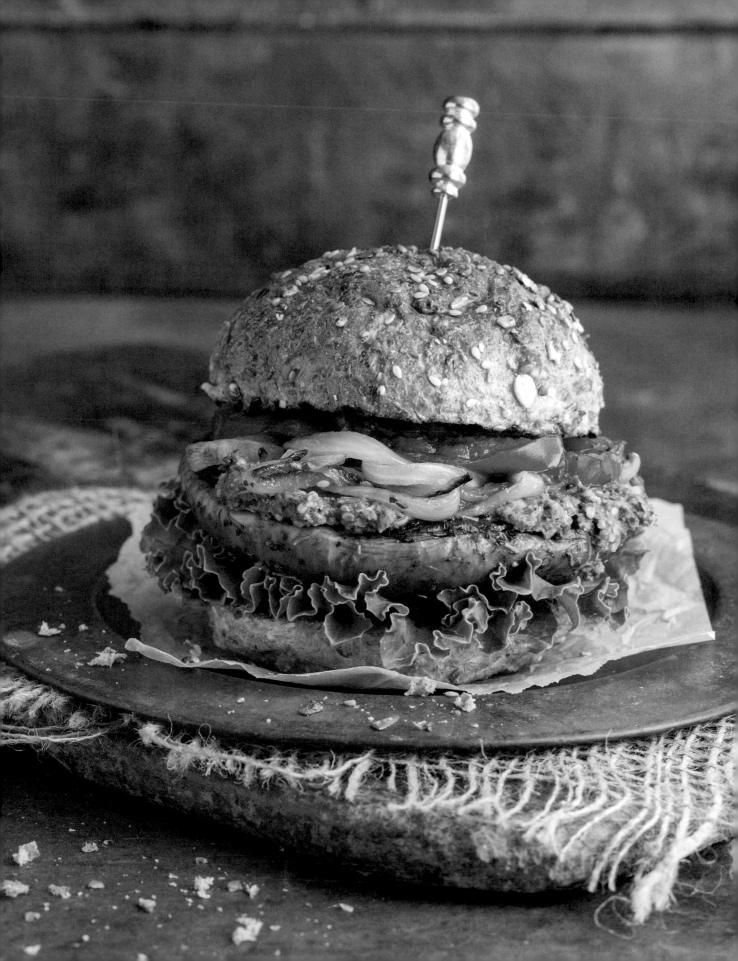

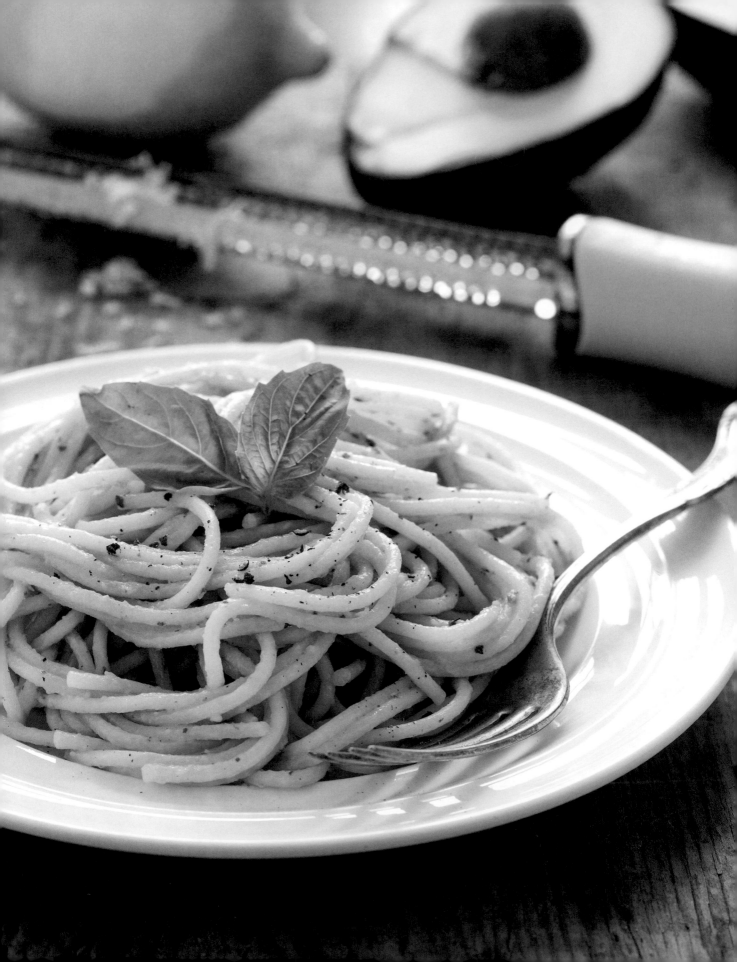

15-minute creamy avocado pasta

255g uncooked pasta (use gluten-free, if desired)

1 to 2 cloves garlic, to taste

10g fresh basil leaves, plus more for serving

4 to 6 teaspoons fresh lemon juice, to taste

1 tablespoon extra-virgin olive oil

1 ripe medium avocado, pitted

¼ to ½ teaspoon fine-grain sea salt

Freshly ground black pepper

Lemon zest, for serving

Praised for how easy it is to prepare and for its dairy-free avocado cream sauce, this recipe is one of the most beloved on my website. Heart-healthy avocados are processed with garlic, a touch of olive oil, fresh basil, lemon juice, and sea salt to create one amazing creamy pasta sauce you won't soon forget.

Serves 3

PREP TIME: 5 to 10 minutes • COOK TIME: 8 to 10 minutes
gluten-free, nut-free, soy-free, sugar-free, grain-free option

1. Bring a large pot of salted water to the boil. Cook the pasta according to the instructions on the package.

2. While the pasta cooks, make the sauce: In a food processor, combine the garlic and basil and pulse to mince.

3. Add the lemon juice, oil, avocado flesh, and 1 tablespoon of water and process until smooth, stopping to scrape down the bowl as needed. If the sauce is too thick, add another tablespoon of water. Season with salt and pepper to taste.

4. Drain the pasta and place it back in the pot. Add the avocado sauce and stir until combined. You can gently rewarm the pasta if it has cooled slightly, or simply serve it at room temperature.

5. Top with lemon zest, pepper, and fresh basil leaves, if desired.

Tips: Because avocados oxidize quickly after you slice them, this sauce is best served immediately. If you do have leftover sauce, transfer it to an airtight container and refrigerate for up to 1 day.

For a grain-free version, serve this avocado sauce with spiralized or julienned courgette (see page 23) or on a bed of spaghetti squash.

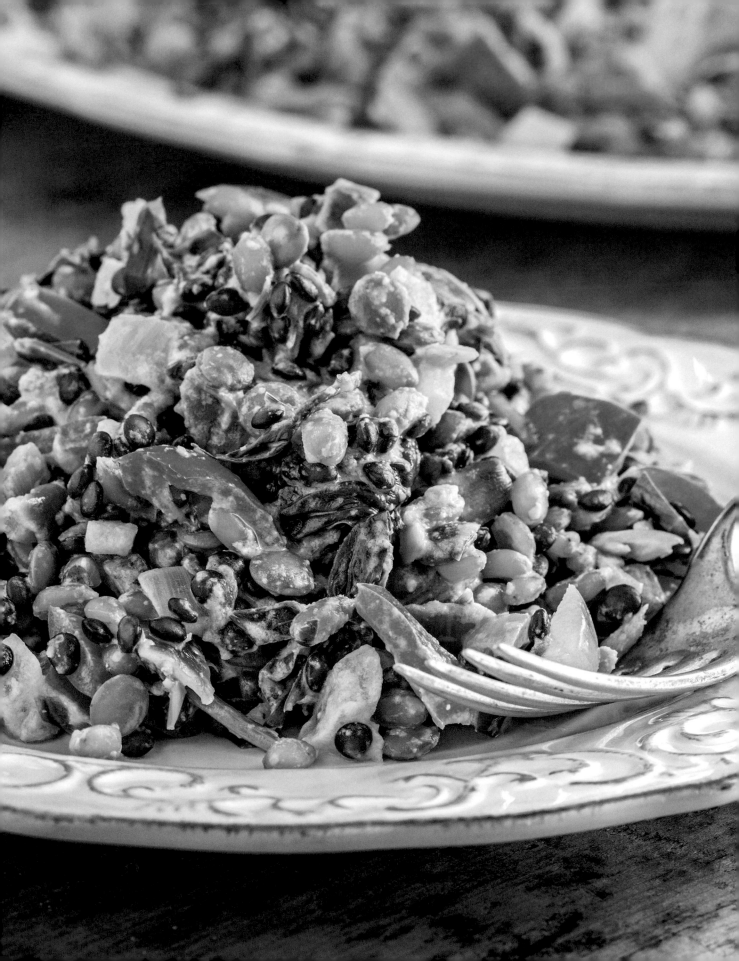

protein power goddess bowl

FOR THE LEMON-TAHINI GODDESS
DRESSING:
60g tahini

1 large clove garlic

125ml fresh lemon juice (from about
2 lemons)

30g nutritional yeast

2 to 3 tablespoons extra-virgin olive oil,
to taste

½ teaspoon fine-grain sea salt,
or to taste, plus more as needed

Freshly ground black pepper

FOR THE LENTIL MIXTURE:
120g uncooked green lentils or a mixture
of green and black lentils

120g uncooked spelt berries or wheat
berries, soaked overnight

1½ teaspoons olive oil

1 small red onion, chopped

3 cloves garlic, minced

1 red bell pepper, chopped

1 large tomato, chopped

220g spinach or lacinato kale, roughly
chopped

10g fresh parsley leaves, minced

This recipe is inspired by one of my favourite vegetarian restaurants, The Coup, in Calgary, Alberta. A rich, tangy lemon-tahini sauce coats chewy lentils and crunchy vegetables. This recipe makes several servings, so it's great if you want leftovers in the fridge for quick grab-and-go meals.

Serves 4 to 6

PREP TIME: 30 minutes

COOK TIME: 50 to 60 minutes

nut-free, soy-free, sugar-free, gluten-free option, grain-free option

1. Make the Lemon-Tahini Goddess Dressing: In a food processor, combine the tahini, garlic, lemon juice, nutritional yeast, extra-virgin olive oil, ½ teaspoon salt, and black pepper to taste and process until smooth. Set aside until ready to use.

2. Cook the lentils according to the instructions on page 302. Set aside.

3. Cook the spelt berries according to the instructions on page 302. Set aside.

4. In a large frying pan, heat the olive oil over a medium heat. Add the onion and garlic and sauté for a few minutes, until the onion is translucent.

5. Add the bell pepper and tomato and sauté for 7 to 8 minutes more, until most of the liquid has cooked off.

6. Stir in the spinach and sauté for a few minutes more, until the greens wilt.

7. Stir in all of the Lemon-Tahini Goddess Dressing and the cooked lentils and spelt berries. Reduce the heat to low and simmer for a

few minutes more. Remove the pan from the heat and stir in the minced parsley.

8. Season with salt and black pepper to taste.

Tips: Looking for a gluten-free version? Use brown rice or quinoa instead of spelt berries.

For a grain-free option, omit the spelt berries.

enlightened miso power bowl

1 sweet potato, cut into 1cm rounds

1½ teaspoons olive oil or coconut oil, melted

Fine-grain sea salt and freshly ground black pepper

170g uncooked quinoa

TO ASSEMBLE:
155g frozen shelled edamame, thawed

1 medium carrot, julienned

2 green onions, thinly sliced

10g fresh coriander leaves, chopped

1 teaspoon sesame seeds (optional)

1 tablespoon hemp seeds (optional)

15g sprouts (optional)

Orange-Maple Miso Dressing (see page 153)

This is a fun power bowl recipe that will keep your energy high for hours. Miso is a fermented food that aids in digestion and adds a wonderful umami flavour to foods. If you are new to miso, Orange-Maple Miso Dressing is a great way to incorporate it into your diet.

Serves 2

PREP TIME: 20 minutes

COOK TIME: 28 to 30 minutes

gluten-free, nut-free, refined sugar-free, soy-free option

1. Preheat the oven to 200°C (400°F). Line a large rimmed baking sheet with parchment paper. Place the sweet potato rounds on the prepared baking sheet and drizzle them with the oil, rubbing it on both sides to coat. Sprinkle the sweet potatoes with salt and pepper. Roast for 20 minutes, then flip the potatoes and roast for 8 to 10 minutes more, until tender and lightly browned.

2. Meanwhile, cook the quinoa following the instructions on page 302.

3. To assemble, divide the cooked quinoa evenly between 2 plates or bowls and season it with salt and pepper. Top with the roasted sweet potato rounds, the edamame, carrots, green onion, coriander, and, if using, the sesame seeds, hemp seeds, and sprouts. Drizzle with Orange-Maple Miso Dressing and enjoy!

Tips: Keep the dressing separate from the salad until just before serving, otherwise it will soak into the quinoa and the flavours will be subdued.

For a soy-free option, omit the edamame and use a soy-free miso, such as South River chickpea miso.

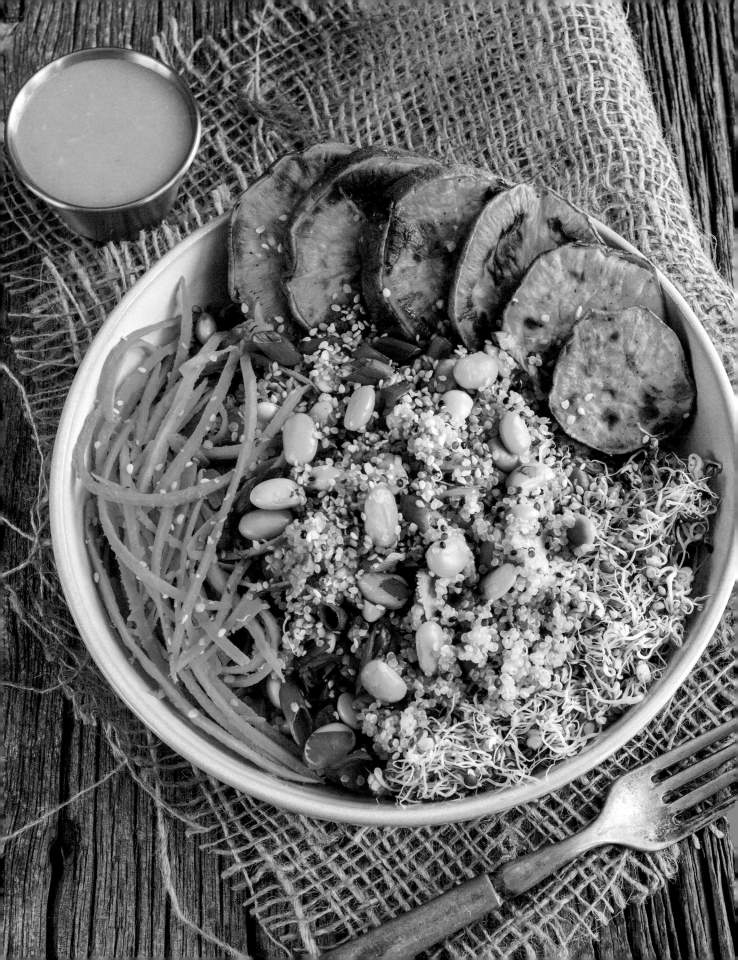

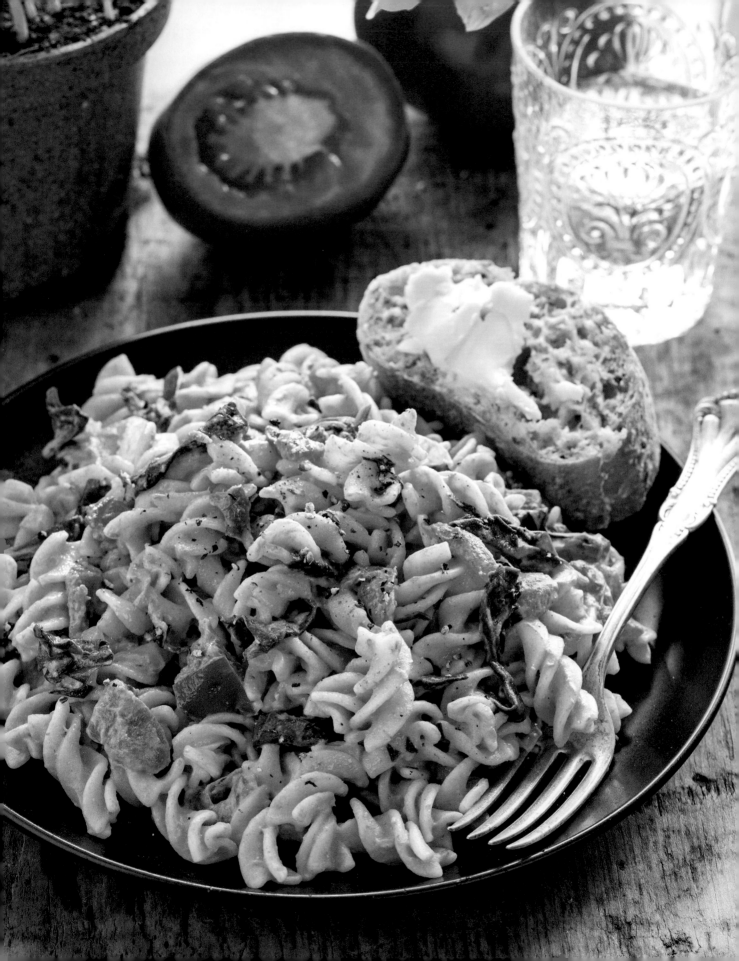

luxurious tomato-basil pasta

75g raw cashews

125ml unsweetened, unflavoured almond milk

255g uncooked pasta (use gluten-free, if desired)

1 teaspoon extra-virgin olive oil

1 small onion, diced

2 cloves garlic, minced

300g diced fresh or canned tomatoes (drain juice, if using canned)

3 handfuls spinach

1 to 3 tablespoons nutritional yeast, to taste (optional)

20g packed fresh basil, finely chopped

2 to 3 tablespoons tomato paste, to taste

1 teaspoon dried oregano

½ teaspoon fine-grain sea salt, or to taste

¼ teaspoon freshly ground black pepper, or to taste

Tip: If at any point the sauce or pasta dries out, just stir in an extra splash of unsweetened, unflavoured almond milk to moisten.

This is one of my husband's favourite meals and he prepares it often while exclaiming, 'It's so easy, even I can make a gourmet dish!' It's the cream sauce, made from raw soaked cashews, that takes this traditional tomato basil pasta to a new level. If you are tired of regular red sauce, try this version for a change. Just be warned – you might never go back!

Serves 3

PREP TIME: 20 minutes • COOK TIME: 30 minutes

gluten-free option, soy-free, sugar-free

1. Place the cashews in a bowl and add enough water to cover. Soak the cashews for at least 2 hours, or overnight. Drain and rinse the cashews. Place them in a blender along with the almond milk and blend on the highest speed until smooth. Set aside.

2. Bring a large pot of salted water to the boil. Prepare the pasta according to the instructions on the package, cooking until al dente.

3. In a large wok, heat the oil over a medium heat. Add the onion and garlic and sauté for 5 to 10 minutes, or until the onion is translucent. Add the diced tomatoes and spinach and continue cooking for 7 to 10 minutes over a medium-high heat, until the spinach is wilted.

4. Stir in the cashew cream, nutritional yeast (if using), basil, tomato paste, oregano, salt, and pepper, and cook for 5 to 10 minutes more, or until heated through.

5. Drain the pasta and add it to the wok. Stir to combine the pasta with the sauce. Cook for a few minutes, or until heated through. Season with salt and pepper to taste and serve immediately.

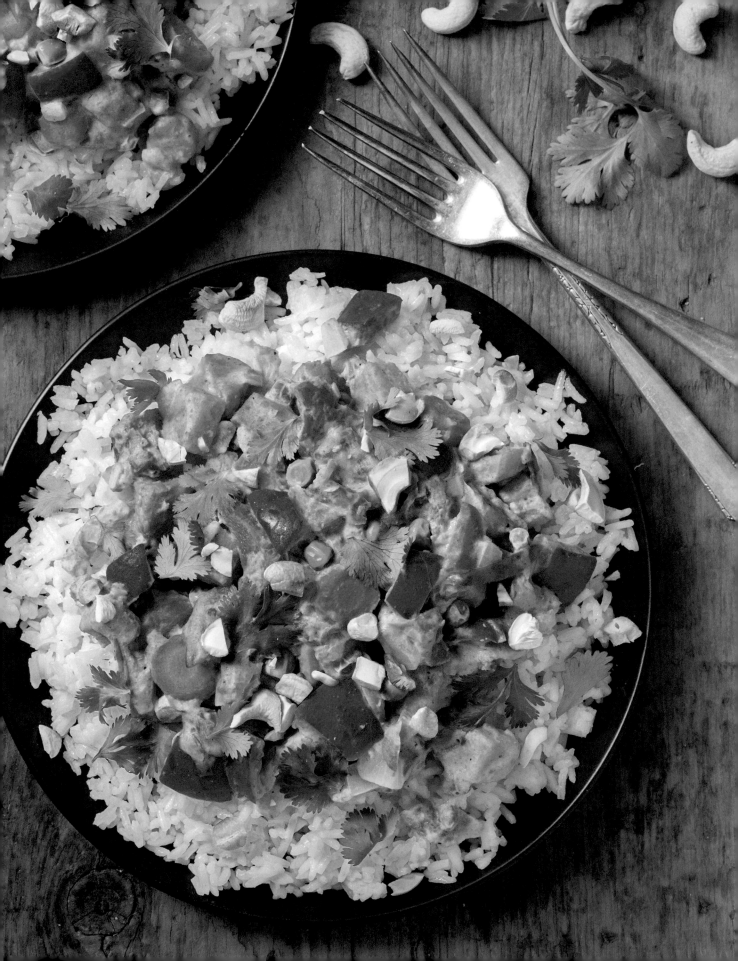

creamy vegetable curry

75g raw cashews, soaked (see page 11)

1 tablespoon coconut oil

1 small onion, diced

3 cloves garlic, minced

1½ teaspoons grated peeled fresh ginger

1 green chilli or jalapeño, seeded, if desired, and diced (optional)

2 medium yellow potatoes or 1 medium sweet potato, peeled and diced

2 medium carrots, diced

1 red bell pepper, chopped

1 large tomato, seeded and chopped

2 tablespoons mild yellow curry powder, or to taste

½ to ¾ teaspoon fine-grain sea salt, plus more as needed

150g frozen or fresh peas

Basmati rice, for serving (optional)

Fresh coriander leaves, for serving

Toasted cashews, for serving

Tip: For a grain-free option, omit the basmati rice.

When I dream of comfort food, I dream of this mild vegetable curry. The rich cream sauce made from soaked raw cashews is balanced with a heavy hand of vegetables. This recipe is versatile and can be made with a variety of different vegetables – broccoli, cauliflower, and sweet potatoes would all be good ones to try. To make it even heartier, serve this over a bed of long-grain rice, such as basmati, or to boost the protein, try adding tofu. This is a lightly spiced and generally mild dish, so if you are a fan of spicy food, use a hot curry powder to heat things up. Be sure to soak the cashews overnight, or for at least three to four hours, so they're ready when you need them.

Serves 4

PREP TIME: 25 minutes • COOK TIME: 25 minutes

gluten-free, soy-free, sugar-free, grain-free option

1. In a blender, combine the cashews with 175ml of water and blend until smooth and creamy. Set aside.

2. In a large frying pan, heat the oil over medium heat. Add the onion, garlic, and ginger and sauté for about 5 minutes, until the onion is translucent. Stir in the green chilli (if using), potatoes, carrots, bell pepper, tomato, curry powder, and salt. Sauté for 5 minutes more.

3. Stir in the cashew cream and peas. Reduce the heat to medium-low and cover the pan with a lid. Simmer, covered, over a medium heat for about 20 minutes, or until the potatoes are fork-tender. Stir every 5 minutes throughout the cooking process. If the mixture starts to dry out, reduce the heat and add a splash of water or oil and stir to combine.

4. Serve the curry over a bed of basmati rice, if desired, and sprinkle with coriander leaves and toasted cashews.

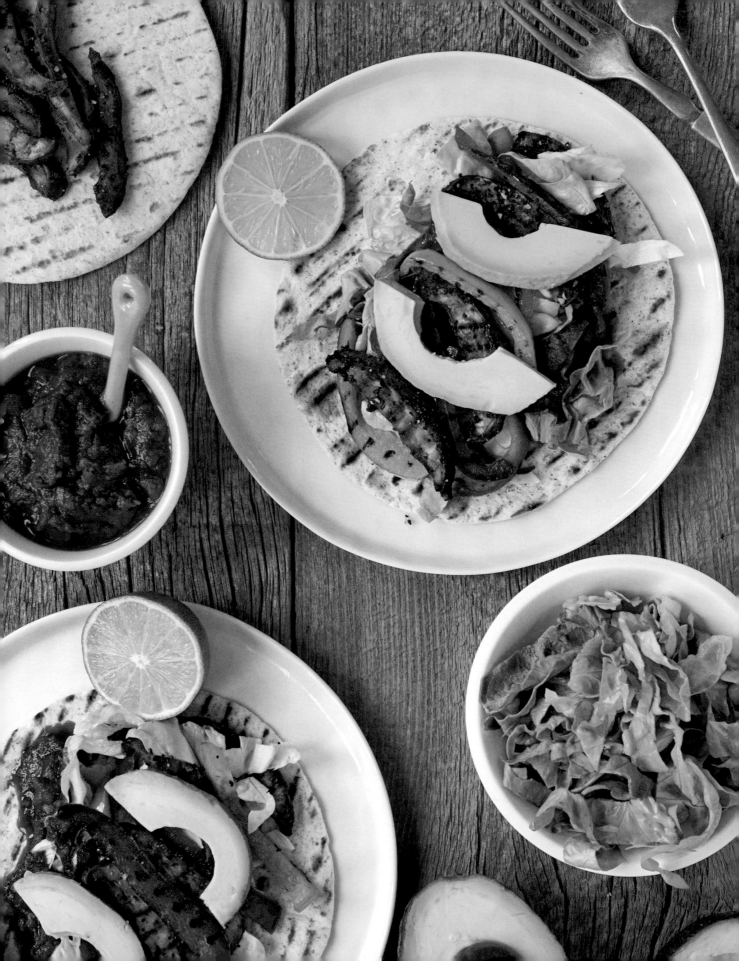

portobello 'steak' fajitas

FOR THE PORTOBELLO STEAKS:

4 to 6 large portobello mushrooms
(450g to 565g)

2 tablespoons plus 1½ teaspoons
grapeseed oil

2 tablespoons fresh lime juice

1 teaspoon dried oregano

1 teaspoon ground cumin

¾ teaspoon chilli powder

½ teaspoon fine-grain sea salt

Freshly ground black pepper

FOR THE STIR-FRY:

1 tablespoon grapeseed, olive, or
coconut oil

1 large red bell pepper, thinly sliced

1 large orange bell pepper, thinly sliced

1 medium yellow onion, thinly sliced

TO ASSEMBLE:

4 to 6 small flour tortillas or lettuce leaves,
for wrapping

Sliced avocado

Cashew Cream (see page 281)

Salsa

Fresh lime juice

Hot sauce

Coriander

Shredded lettuce

When you marinate portobello mushrooms and season them with taco spices, you can make a fantastic meatless filling for fajitas or tacos. My husband, who isn't a big fan of mushrooms, absolutely loves these fajitas, probably because he can go wild with all the toppings and create something new each time. If we want a lighter meal in the summer, we'll often use lettuce wraps in place of flour tortillas, so keep this in mind for a gluten-free and grain-free option. You can also use corn tortillas.

Makes 4 to 6 fajitas

PREP TIME: 30 minutes • COOK TIME: 20 to 25 minutes

gluten-free option, sugar-free, soy-free, grain-free option

1. Make the Portobello Steaks: Remove the stems from the portobello mushrooms by twisting the stem until it pops off. Discard the stems or reserve them for another use, such as a stir-fry. With a small spoon, scrape out and discard the inside black gills from the mushroom caps. Rub the mushroom caps with a damp cloth to remove any debris. Slice them into long, 1cm-wide strips.

2. In a large bowl, whisk together the oil, lime juice, oregano, cumin, chilli powder, salt, and pepper to taste. Add the sliced mushrooms and toss well to coat. Let the mushrooms marinate for 20 to 30 minutes, tossing every 10 minutes or so.

3. Meanwhile, make the Stir-fry: In a large frying pan, heat the oil over a medium heat. Add the bell peppers and onion and sauté over a medium-high heat for about 10 minutes, or until the vegetables are softened.

4. Preheat a grill pan over a medium or high heat. Lay the marinated mushrooms on the pan and grill them for 3 to 5 minutes per side, or until they have nice char lines. You can also lightly grill the tortillas, if desired.

5. To assemble, place a tortilla on a plate and top with some of the grilled portobello strips, sautéed vegetables, and your desired toppings. Repeat with the remaining tortillas and toppings. Or, let your guests top their own tortillas. Enjoy!

Tip: For an alternative to mushrooms, you can try my lentil-walnut 'meat' mixture: In a food processor, combine 1 clove garlic, 180g cooked lentils, 125g toasted walnuts, 1½ teaspoons dried oregano, 1½ teaspoons ground cumin, 1½ teaspoons chilli powder, ½ teaspoon fine-grain sea salt, 4 to 6 teaspoons oil, and 2 tablespoons water and pulse until combined and crumbly.

oh she glows

sides

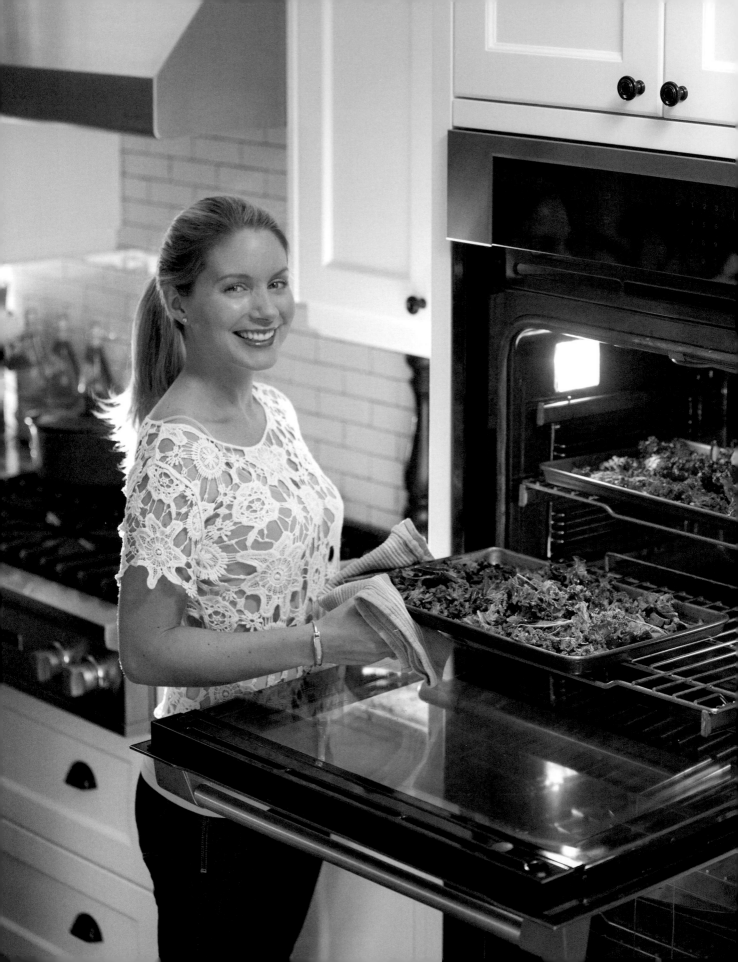

Side dishes are often the unsung heroes of a plant-based diet. I can't tell you how many times I've eaten at non-vegan-friendly restaurants and had to pull together a meal based on simple side dishes like sautéed mushrooms, brown rice, and beans. My dining companions often look at me with sympathy and big sad eyes, but what they don't know is that I often eat this way at home!

Making a simple plant-based meal doesn't have to be fussy; sometimes it just involves pulling a few sides together to create a balanced, nourishing meal. For easy dinners, I try to include a high-protein source, such as my all-time favourite, Marinated Balsamic, Maple & Garlic Tempeh (page 199) or my Pan-Seared Garlic Tofu (page 197), and serve it alongside a grain, such as brown rice, and vegetables, like my Perfect Kale Chips (page 201) or Marinated Italian Mushrooms (page 193). I like to prepare grains ahead of time and freeze them for quick weeknight meal additions. It doesn't get much easier than grabbing a bag of cooked grains from the freezer and reheating it in simmering water or a frying pan. If you are looking for something to serve alongside a veggie burger, try my Perfect Kale Chips or Lightened-Up Crispy Baked Fries (page 203). For cool-weather sides, try Cauliflower Mashed Potatoes with Easy Mushroom Gravy (page 207) or Fall Harvest Butternut Squash with Almond-Pecan Parmesan (page 209). Whatever you're looking for, you'll find something in this chapter for many different occasions.

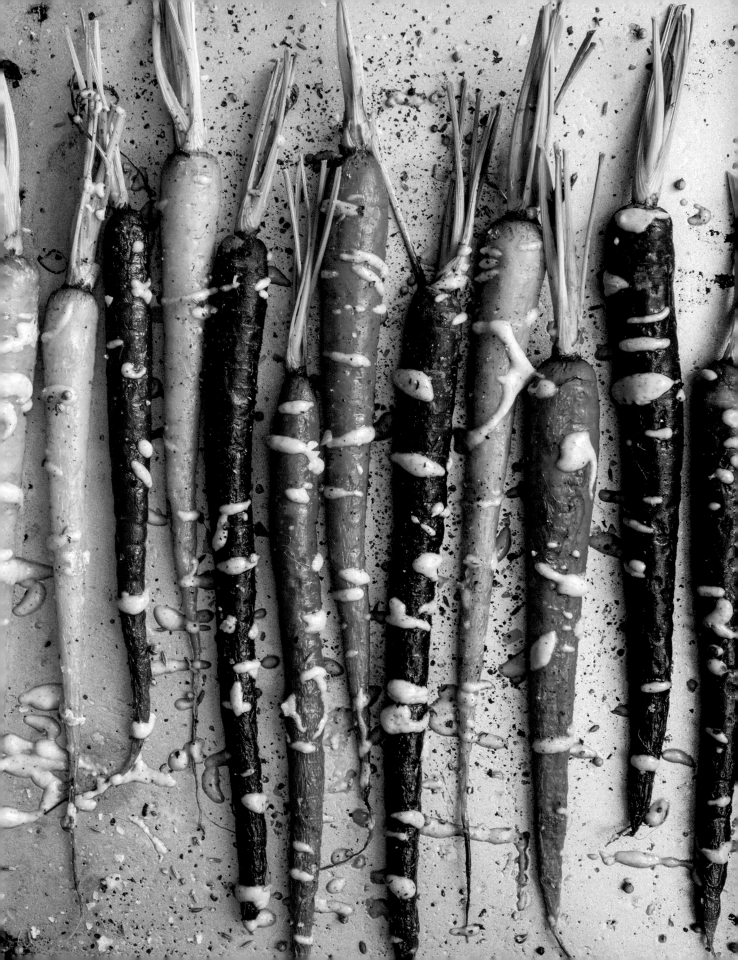

roasted rainbow carrots
with cumin-coriander tahini sauce

FOR THE ROASTED RAINBOW
CARROTS:

2 bunches rainbow carrots (790g)

1 tablespoon grapeseed oil

¾ teaspoon fine-grain sea salt

½ teaspoon cumin seeds

½ teaspoon coriander seeds

¼ teaspoon freshly ground black pepper

FOR THE CUMIN-CORIANDER TAHINI
SAUCE:

2 tablespoons tahini

4 teaspoons fresh lemon juice

1 tablespoon extra-virgin olive oil

1 teaspoon ground cumin

½ teaspoon ground coriander

¼ teaspoon fine-grain sea salt

Rainbow carrots have to be among the most gorgeous vegetables out there. Purple, yellow, orange, and red; it's always amazing that these colours exist in nature, no food dyes required. In this recipe, I've roasted rainbow carrots with cumin and coriander seeds in a bit of oil and salt and then topped them with a delicious lemon-tahini sauce. This is easily my favourite way to enjoy a fresh bunch of spring carrots, and I've been known to polish off an entire batch on my own. Don't worry if you can't find rainbow carrots – regular carrots will work just fine, too.

Serves 4

PREP TIME: 10 minutes • COOK TIME: 15 to 20 minutes

gluten-free, nut-free, soy-free, sugar-free, grain-free

1. Make the Roasted Rainbow Carrots: Preheat the oven to 220°C (425°F). Line a rimmed baking sheet with parchment paper.

2. Trim the stems off the carrots, leaving a couple of inches of the stem intact. Wash the carrots and gently pat them dry.

3. Place the carrots on the prepared baking sheet.

4. Drizzle the carrots with the oil and roll them on the baking sheet until the oil is evenly dispersed. Sprinkle them with the salt, cumin and coriander seed, and pepper. Leave 1cm between each carrot.

5. Roast the carrots for 15 to 20 minutes, or until they are just fork-tender but still a bit firm. Be sure not to overcook them.

6. Make the Cumin-Coriander Tahini Sauce: In a small bowl, whisk together the tahini, lemon juice, oil, cumin, coriander, and salt.

7. Plate the carrots and drizzle the sauce on top. Serve any leftover sauce on the side.

Tip: I usually don't bother peeling rainbow carrots as their skin is quite delicate and thin. However, if you are using regular, pre-trimmed carrots – depending on their size and thickness – you might want to peel them before roasting.

marinated italian mushrooms

900g cremini or white button mushrooms (look for small mushrooms, if possible)

4 tablespoons extra-virgin olive oil

2 large cloves garlic, minced

100g thinly sliced shallots (from about 3 shallots)

10g fresh flat-leaf parsley, chopped

½ teaspoon dried thyme

½ teaspoon dried oregano

¼ teaspoon fine-grain sea salt

¼ teaspoon freshly ground black pepper

3 to 4 tablespoons balsamic vinegar, to taste

I spent the first twenty-five years of my life thinking that I despised mushrooms, only to find out later on that I absolutely adore them. Well, I'm certainly making up for lost time! Not only are mushrooms packed with cancer-fighting nutrients, but they are a satisfying, meaty addition to any plant-based diet. Marinated mushrooms are fairly quick to throw together, and they taste better and better the longer they marinate. I realize two pounds of mushrooms seems like an awful lot, but keep in mind that they reduce in size significantly as they cook down. If you are anything like me, you'll wonder how they disappeared so quickly!

Serves 3 to 4
PREP TIME: 10 to 15 minutes
COOK TIME: 10 to 15 minutes
gluten-free, nut-free, soy-free, sugar-free, grain-free

1. Remove the stems from the mushrooms by twisting the stem until it pops off. Discard the stems or reserve them for another use, such as a stir-fry. Gently rub the mushroom caps with a damp cloth to remove any debris.

2. In a large wok, heat 2 tablespoons of the oil over medium heat. Add the garlic and shallots and sauté for 2 to 3 minutes. Raise the heat to medium-high and add the mushroom caps. Sauté, stirring frequently, for 7 to 8 minutes more.

3. With a slotted spoon, transfer the mushroom mixture to a large bowl, discarding the leftover water and oil in the wok. Stir in the parsley, thyme, oregano, salt, pepper, vinegar, and remaining 2 tablespoons oil until combined.

4. Let the mushrooms cool for 20 to 30 minutes, then cover the bowl and refrigerate for at least 2 hours, or overnight, so the flavours can develop. I try to stir the mushrooms a few times during this process.

5. Serve the mushrooms chilled or at room temperature.

....
oh she glows

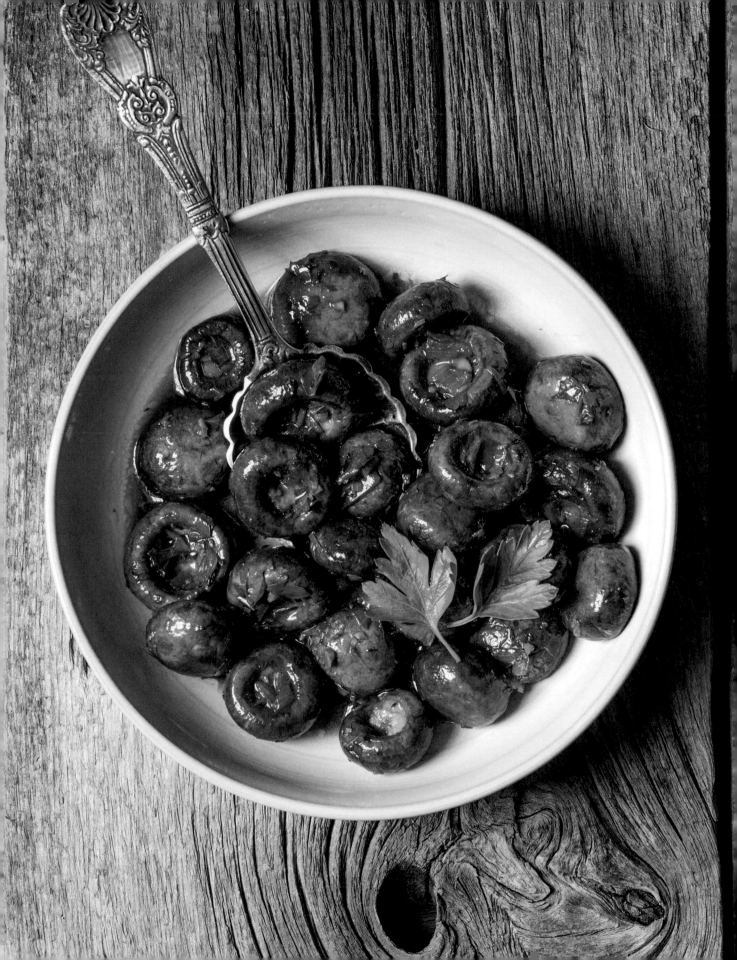

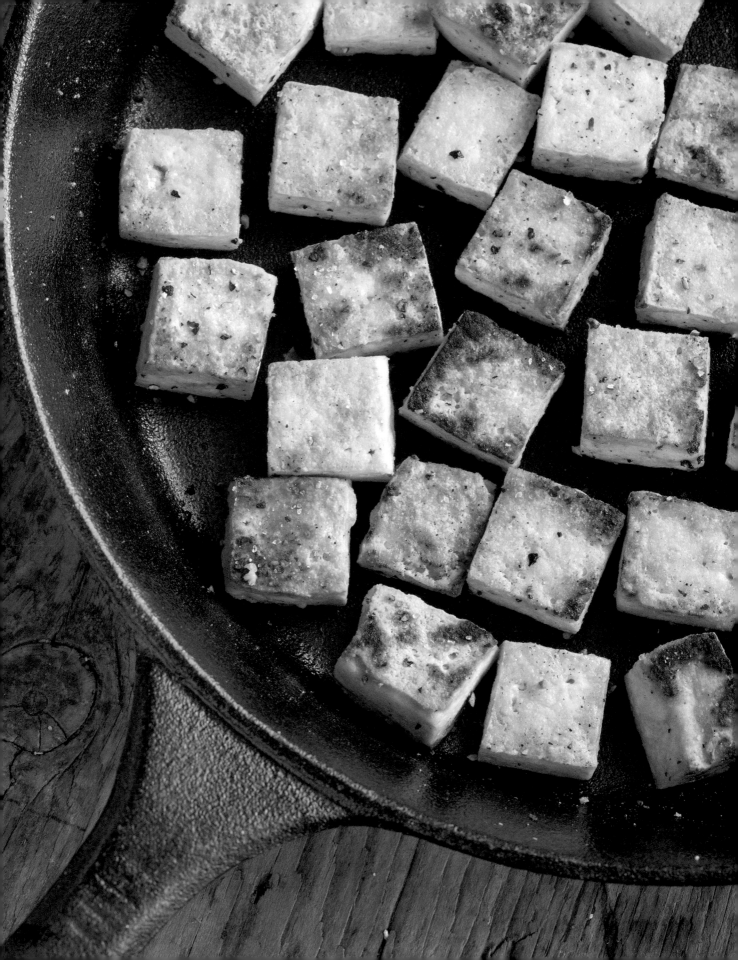

pan-seared garlic tofu

1 454g block firm or extra-firm tofu

1 teaspoon garlic powder

¼ teaspoon fine-grain sea salt

¼ teaspoon freshly ground
black pepper

1 tablespoon melted coconut oil, or
grapeseed oil

This method will give you crispy, lightly seasoned pan-fried tofu without the need for much oil. Use a cast-iron skillet if you have one to hand, as it will intensify the crispy shell of the tofu (a regular skillet will work just fine, too).

Serves 4

PREP TIME: 5 to 10 minutes • COOK TIME: 6 to 10 minutes

gluten-free, nut-free, sugar-free, grain-free

1. Following the instructions on page 285, press the tofu overnight, or for at least 25 to 30 minutes.

2. Slice the pressed tofu into 9 to 10 1cm-thick rectangles and then slice each rectangle into 6 squares, to make a total of 54 to 60 tofu pieces.

3. Preheat a cast-iron skillet (or regular skillet) over a medium-high heat for several minutes.

4. In a large bowl, combine the tofu squares, garlic powder, salt, and pepper and toss until fully coated.

5. When a drop of water sizzles on the skillet, it's ready. Add the oil and tilt the skillet to coat it evenly with the oil. Carefully add the tofu to the pan (be careful, as the oil might splatter; use a splatter guard if needed) in a single layer, making sure all the pieces lay flat against the skillet.

6. Cook the tofu for 3 to 5 minutes, until a golden crust forms. Flip each piece and cook for 3 to 5 minutes more, until golden. Serve immediately.

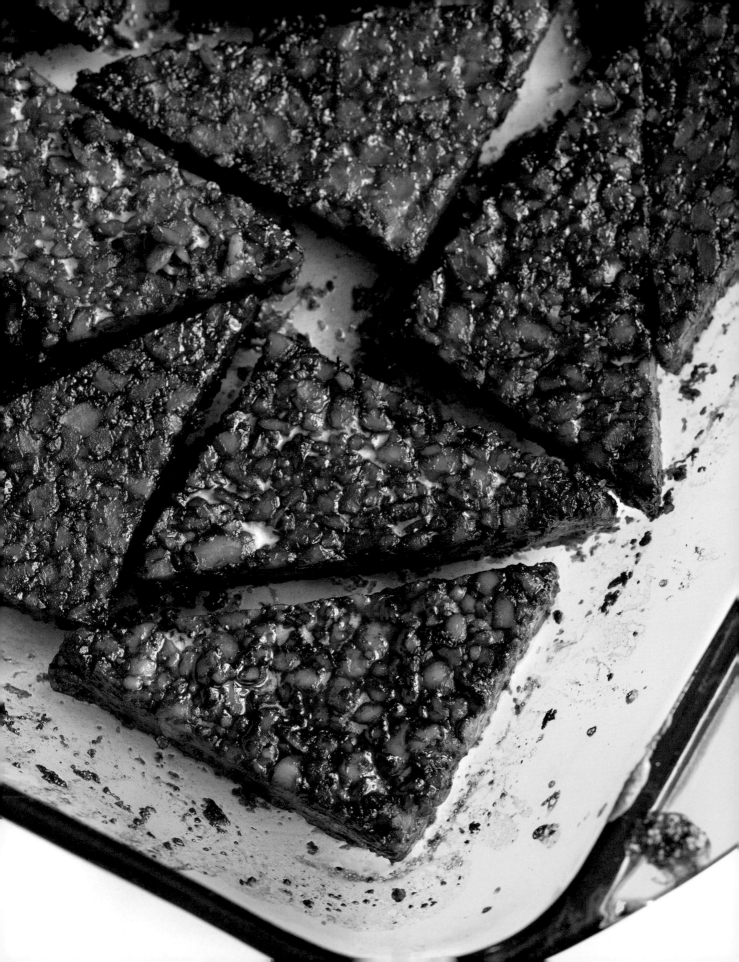

marinated balsamic, maple & garlic tempeh

1 240g package tempeh

125ml balsamic vinegar

2 cloves garlic, minced

4 teaspoons low-sodium tamari

1 tablespoon pure maple syrup

1 tablespoon extra-virgin olive oil

I thought I didn't like tempeh. I thought it wasn't for me. After a few unsuccessful attempts at trying desperately to like tempeh, I almost crossed it off my list forever. This recipe, however, changed everything and instantly made tempeh a new favorite in my diet. A special thanks to my friend Meghan Telpner, who blogs at meghantelpner.com, for inspiring this delectable recipe! If you've ever had a bad experience with tempeh, I urge you (no, beg you!) to give this recipe a try. It just might change your life!

Serves 3

PREP TIME: 5 minutes

MARINATE TIME: 2 hours or overnight

COOK TIME: 30 to 35 minutes

gluten-free, nut-free, refined sugar-free

1. Rinse the tempeh and pat dry. Slice the tempeh into 8 thin (1cm) pieces, then halve them on the diagonal to make a total of 16 triangles. Or simply slice them into any shape you wish.

2. In a large glass baking dish, whisk together the balsamic vinegar, minced garlic, tamari, maple syrup, and oil.

3. Add the tempeh to the dish and gently toss to coat with the marinade. Cover the dish with foil and marinate the tempeh in the refrigerator for at least 2 hours, or overnight, gently tossing the tempeh every now and then.

4. Preheat the oven to 180°C (350°F).

5. Spread the marinated tempeh triangles in a single layer in the baking dish and cover with foil. Bake the tempeh in the marinade for 15 minutes. Remove the foil and flip the tempeh in the marinade. Bake, uncovered, for 15 to 20 minutes more, until the tempeh has absorbed most of the marinade.

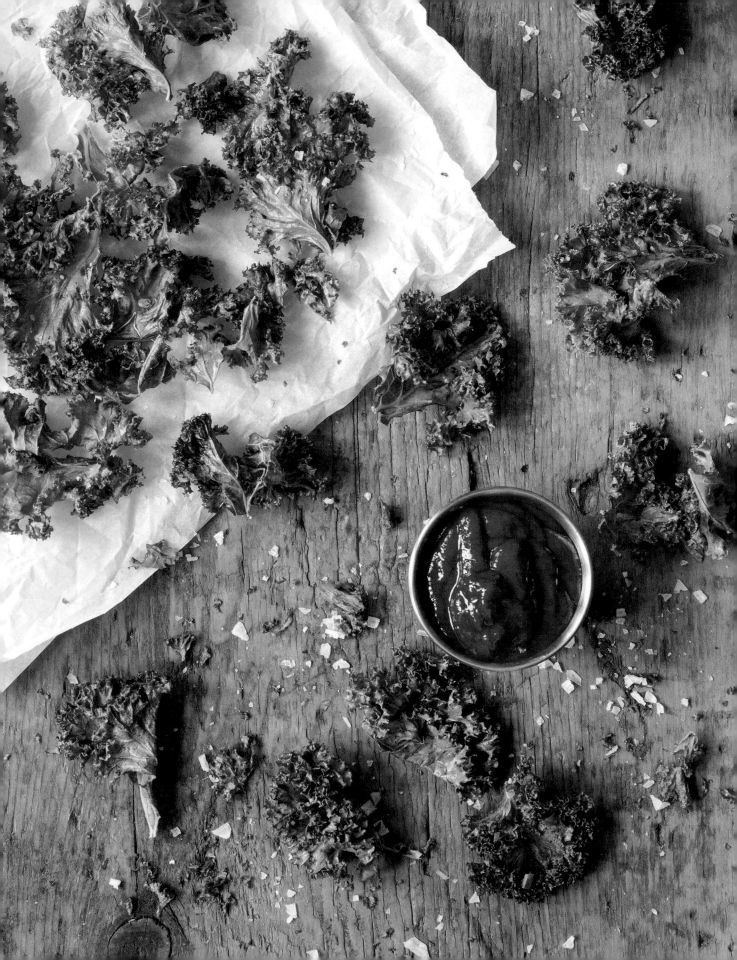

perfect kale chips

1 bunch kale, stems removed and leaves torn (see Tip, page 122)

1 tablespoon extra-virgin olive oil

¼ to ½ teaspoon fine-grain sea salt

¼ teaspoon freshly ground black pepper

Spices or seasonings of choice (optional)

Ketchup, sriracha, or salad dressing, for dipping

Tip: If you are new to kale chips, it can take some time before they grow on you. Give them an honest try, and I promise that in due time, they will grow on you like a (superfood) weed.

After testing several kale chip recipes that were hit-and-miss, I made it my mission to bake the perfect chip for this book. I tested all different kinds of oven temperatures – from high to ultra-low heat, and I found that baking at a lower temperature (150°C/300°F) for a slightly longer time yielded the best result. When you cook at a lower temperature, you aren't left with unevenly baked kale chips (and the dreaded burned ones!). Feel free to sprinkle on your favourite spices and seasonings before baking. I love these with just a little olive oil, garlic, and sea salt, and I dip them in some organic ketchup if I want something sweet. If you've ever been discouraged by a bad batch of kale chips, I encourage you to give this recipe a try.

Serves 3

PREP TIME: 5 to 10 minutes   •   COOK TIME: 17 to 20 minutes

gluten-free, nut-free, soy-free, sugar-free

1. Preheat the oven to 150°C (300°F). Line two large rimmed baking sheets with parchment paper. Wash the kale leaves and dry them completely in a salad spinner.

2. Place the kale leaves in a large bowl and drizzle with the oil. Massage the oil into the kale with your hands until the leaves are thoroughly coated with the oil.

3. Place the kale in a single layer on the prepared baking sheets. Sprinkle with salt, pepper, and other spices or seasonings, if desired. Bake for 10 minutes, then rotate the pans and bake for 7 to 10 minutes more, until the leaves are crispy but not burned. Serve the kale chips with a side of ketchup, sriracha, or your favourite salad dressing. Leftover kale chips don't keep their crispiness very well, so these are best consumed immediately. I usually just leave them on the pan and pick away at them all day long!

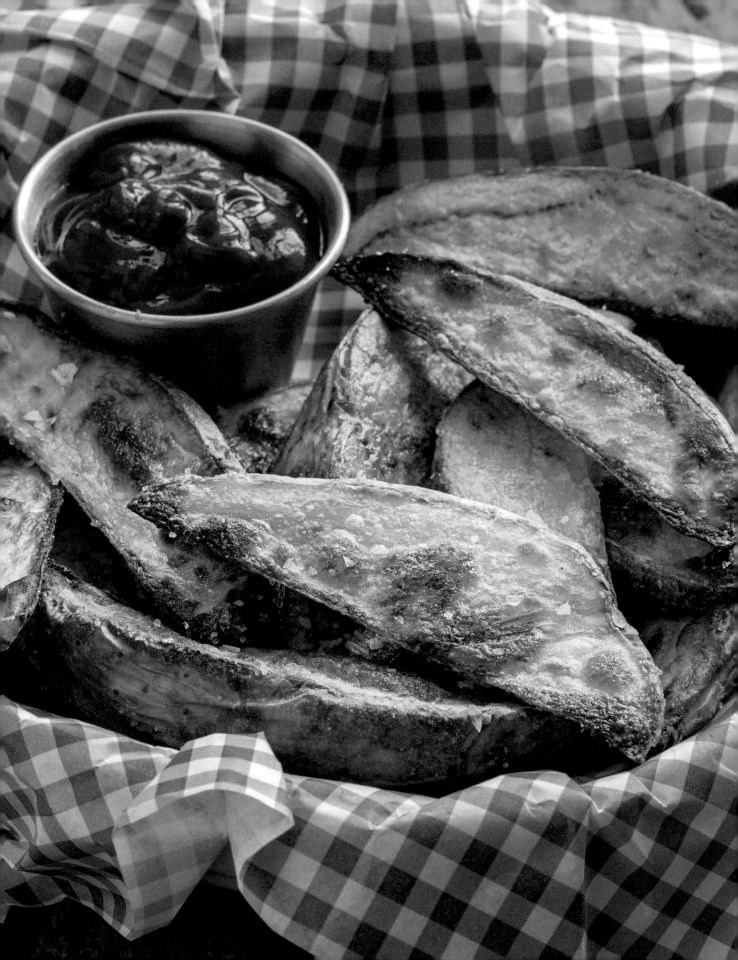

lightened-up crispy baked fries

2 large Yukon Gold potatoes
(about 450g)

1 tablespoon arrowroot powder

1 tablespoon grapeseed oil

½ teaspoon fine-grain sea salt

Freshly ground black pepper

Seasonings (such as garlic powder,
chilli powder, etc.), if desired

It takes just five to ten minutes to prep a couple of potatoes and turn them into delicious, crispy baked fries. This method of making fries forgoes frying and instead calls for roasting the potatoes in a light coating of arrowroot powder and oil. The resulting fries are perfectly crispy and lightly golden brown. Try pairing them with Our Favourite Veggie Burger (see page 155) for a meal that's sure to impress.

Serves 2

PREP TIME: 10 minutes • COOK TIME: 30 to 35 minutes
gluten-free, nut-free, soy-free, sugar-free, grain-free

1. Preheat the oven to 220°C (425°F). Line a rimmed baking sheet with parchment paper.

2. Quarter the potatoes lengthwise. Slice each quarter in half (or into thirds, if the potatoes are very large).

3. Place the arrowroot powder and potato wedges in a small kitchen garbage bag. Twist the top of the bag closed securely and shake the bag vigorously until the potatoes are coated with the powder.

4. Drizzle the oil into the bag, twist it closed again, and shake until the potatoes are fully coated. I know it sounds weird, but it works!

5. Place the potatoes on the prepared baking sheet, leaving at least 2cm between them. (Spacing them too close together may result in less crispy fries.) Season with salt and pepper and additional seasonings, if desired.

6. Bake for 15 minutes, then flip the potatoes and bake for 10 to 20 minutes more, until golden and puffy. Serve the fries immediately, as they will lose their crispiness with time.

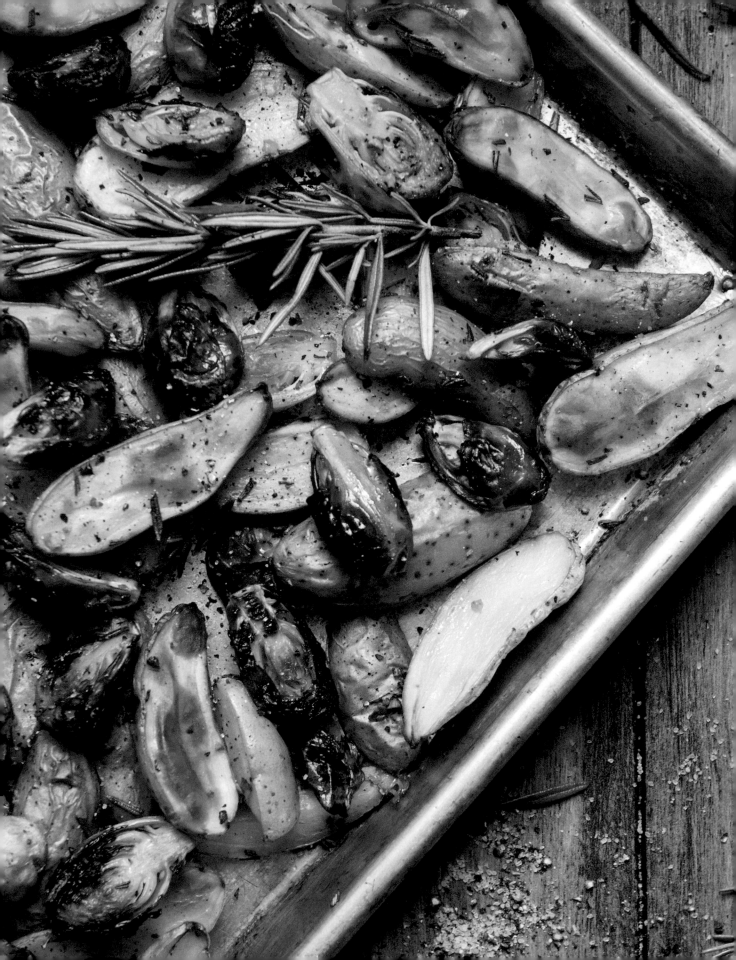

roasted brussels sprouts with fingerling potatoes and rosemary

790g fingerling potatoes

340g Brussels sprouts, trimmed

3 cloves garlic, minced

2 tablespoons minced fresh rosemary

4 teaspoons extra-virgin olive oil

1½ teaspoons Sucanat sugar or other granulated sweetener

¾ teaspoon fine-grain sea salt, plus more as needed

¼ teaspoon freshly ground black pepper, plus more as needed

¼ teaspoon red pepper flakes (optional)

Growing up, I despised Brussels sprouts, as most children do. But in my early twenties, I gave them another shot, and they slowly grew on me over the course of many holiday dinners. I'd place a few on the edge of my plate 'just to try,' and eventually I started to enjoy their meaty texture. Yes, I just combined 'meaty' and 'Brussels sprouts' in the same sentence! This recipe features roasted fingerlings, my most-loved potatoes of all time, with a generous amount of fresh rosemary and garlic and, of course, hearty Brussels sprouts. Try it and see why this recipe has turned many Brussels sprouts haters into glowing fans!

Serves 4 to 5

PREP TIME: 20 minutes • COOK TIME: 35 to 38 minutes

gluten-free, nut-free, soy-free, refined sugar-free, grain-free

1. Preheat the oven to 200°C (400°F). Line a large rimmed baking sheet with parchment paper.

2. Scrub the fingerling potatoes and pat them dry. Halve the potatoes lengthwise and place them in a very large bowl.

3. Trim the stem off the Brussels sprouts and remove loose leaves. Rinse the Brussels sprouts and pat them dry. Slice the Brussels sprouts in half through the stem end and place them in the bowl with the potatoes.

4. Add the garlic, rosemary, oil, sugar, salt, pepper, and red pepper flakes (if using) and stir until the potatoes and Brussels sprouts are coated in the mixture. Transfer the mixture to the prepared baking sheet.

5. Roast for 35 to 38 minutes, stirring once halfway through the baking time, until the potatoes are golden and the Brussels sprouts are lightly charred. Season with more salt and pepper, if desired, and serve immediately.

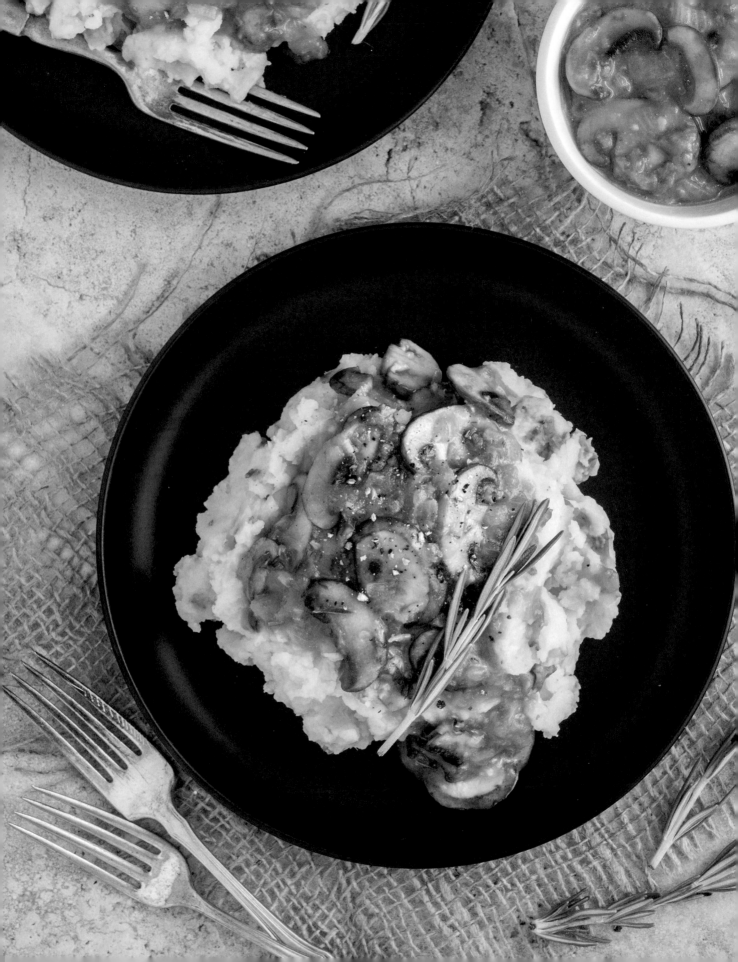

cauliflower mashed potatoes
with easy mushroom gravy

900g Yukon Gold or yellow potatoes, peeled or unpeeled, cut into 2.5cm chunks

1 small head cauliflower (675g), chopped into bite-size florets

2 tablespoons vegan butter

1 teaspoon fine-grain sea salt, or to taste

Freshly ground black pepper

1 clove garlic, minced

Non-dairy milk, if desired

1 recipe Easy Mushroom Gravy (see page 282)

Tip: Feel free to increase the cauliflower-to-potato ratio as you get used to the cauliflower flavour.

This cauliflower mashed potato dish is a fun way to sneak a superfood vegetable into your normal mashed potatoes without anyone being the wiser. When you gently cook cauliflower and mash it into potatoes, you add volume, decrease calories, and, of course, pack in a ton of extra nutrition. I've paired this mash with a rich, yet healthy mushroom gravy, but it's also lovely with a pat of vegan butter. A bit of minced fresh rosemary is great in this, too.

Serves 6

PREP TIME: 30 minutes • COOK TIME: 20 to 30 minutes

gluten-free, nut-free, soy-free, sugar-free, grain-free

1. Place the potatoes in a very large saucepan and add water to cover. Bring the water to the boil and cook the potatoes for 10 minutes, uncovered.

2. After 10 minutes, add the cauliflower to the saucepan with the potatoes. Boil both vegetables for 10 minutes more, uncovered, until they are fork-tender.

3. Drain the potatoes and cauliflower and return them to the saucepan. Mash with a potato masher until smooth, adding the vegan butter and salt, pepper, and garlic as you mash. Resist the urge to add milk right off the bat. As you mash the cauliflower, it will release some water and thin out the mixture. If you need to add some milk at the end, feel free to do so.

4. Serve topped with Easy Mushroom Gravy.

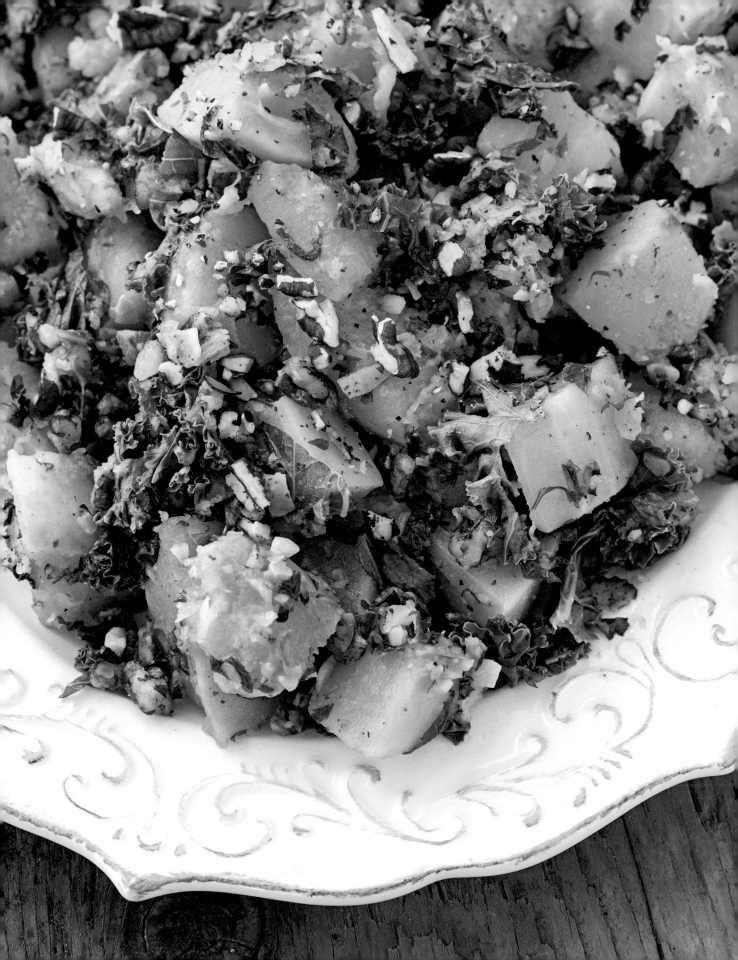

fall harvest butternut squash with almond-pecan parmesan

FOR THE SQUASH:

1 900g to 1.35kg butternut squash, peeled and chopped

2 large cloves garlic, minced

10g fresh parsley leaves, finely chopped

1½ teaspoons extra-virgin olive oil

½ teaspoon fine-grain sea salt

FOR THE ALMOND-PECAN PARMESAN:

35g almonds

35g pecans

1 tablespoon nutritional yeast (optional)

1½ teaspoons extra-virgin olive oil

⅛ teaspoon fine-grain sea salt

225g stemmed chopped lacinato kale leaves

Caramelized roasted butternut squash and thin strips of lacinato kale are topped with toasted Almond-Pecan Parmesan in this delectable fall dish. It's no wonder this comfort food side dish is one of the most popular on my blog. The hardest part about this recipe is chopping up the squash, but it's easy sailing from there. When I'm in a time crunch, I occasionally buy prechopped fresh butternut squash at my local grocery store so I can make this recipe in a heartbeat. Our little secret?

Serves 4

PREP TIME: 30 minutes • COOK TIME: 45 to 55 minutes

gluten-free, soy-free, sugar-free, grain-free

1. Make the Squash: Preheat the oven to 200°C (400°F). Lightly oil a 2.5 to 3l casserole dish.

2. Peel the squash. Thinly slice off the bottom and top and then halve the squash lengthwise. Remove the seeds with a grapefruit spoon or ice-cream scoop. Chop the squash into 2.5cm chunks and place them in the casserole dish.

3. Add the garlic, parsley, oil, and salt and stir until well combined with the squash.

4. Cover the dish with a lid (or foil) and bake for 35 to 40 minutes, or until the squash is fork-tender.

5. Meanwhile, make the Almond-Pecan Parmesan: In a food processor, combine the almonds, pecans, nutritional yeast, oil, and salt and pulse until chunky (or simply chop the nuts by hand and mix everything together in a bowl).

6. When the squash is fork-tender, remove it from the oven and reduce the heat to 180°C (350°F). Carefully fold in the chopped

kale and sprinkle the Almond-Pecan Parmesan all over the squash. Bake for 6 to 8 minutes more, uncovered, until the nuts are lightly toasted and the kale is wilted.

Tip: If you're looking to turn this side dish into a meal, this recipe is fantastic served with Field Roast Smoked Apple Sage sausage.

power snacks

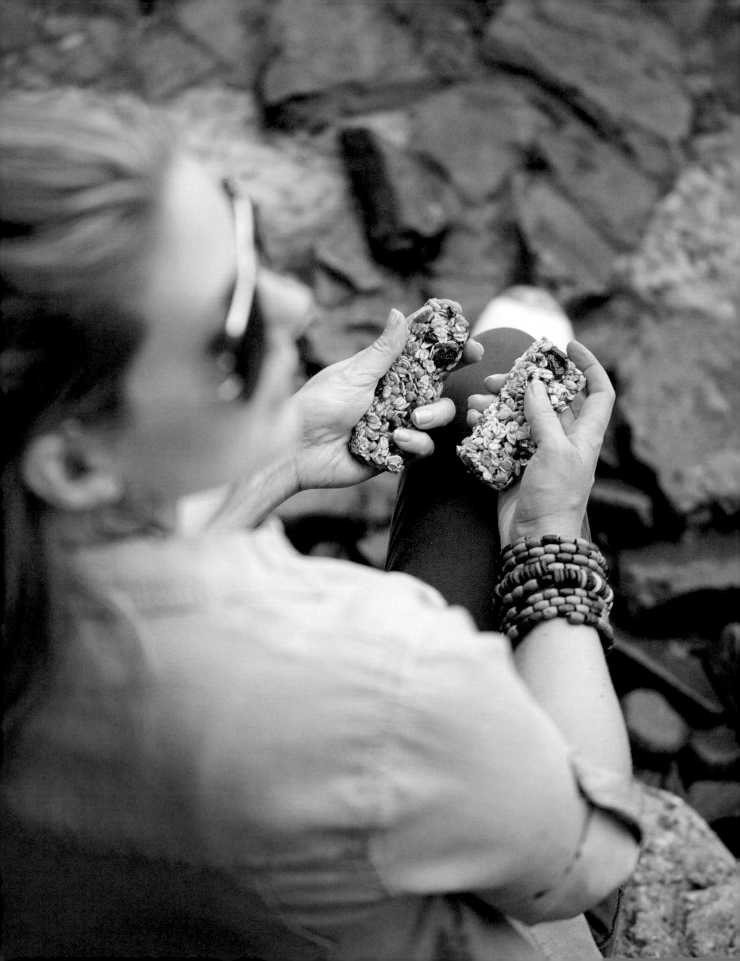

My husband, Eric, can attest to the fact that I'm a much more pleasant person to be around when I have snacks to keep the hunger monster at bay. I'm the girl with the energy bars stashed in her purse at all times, 'just in case.' Once, I found a two-month-old shrivelled-up apple core at the bottom of my purse. Eric just shook his head, obviously not surprised one bit. A snack can often be as simple as an apple with almond butter or hummus and crackers, but when you want to change it up, I hope the recipes in this chapter will inspire you to try something new. In this chapter, you'll also find two of my Glo Bar recipes from the bakery I ran for a couple of years, Glo Bakery. I'm so excited to share these recipes for the first time! Glo Bars make the perfect take-along snack food for gatherings or picnics, and they are great to stock in your freezer for easy snacking. If savoury snacks are more your thing, try my Super-Power Chia Bread (page 229) spread with coconut oil or nut butter or my Perfect Roasted Chickpeas (page 220) if you are in the mood for something crunchy and protein packed. Cheers to healthy snacking!

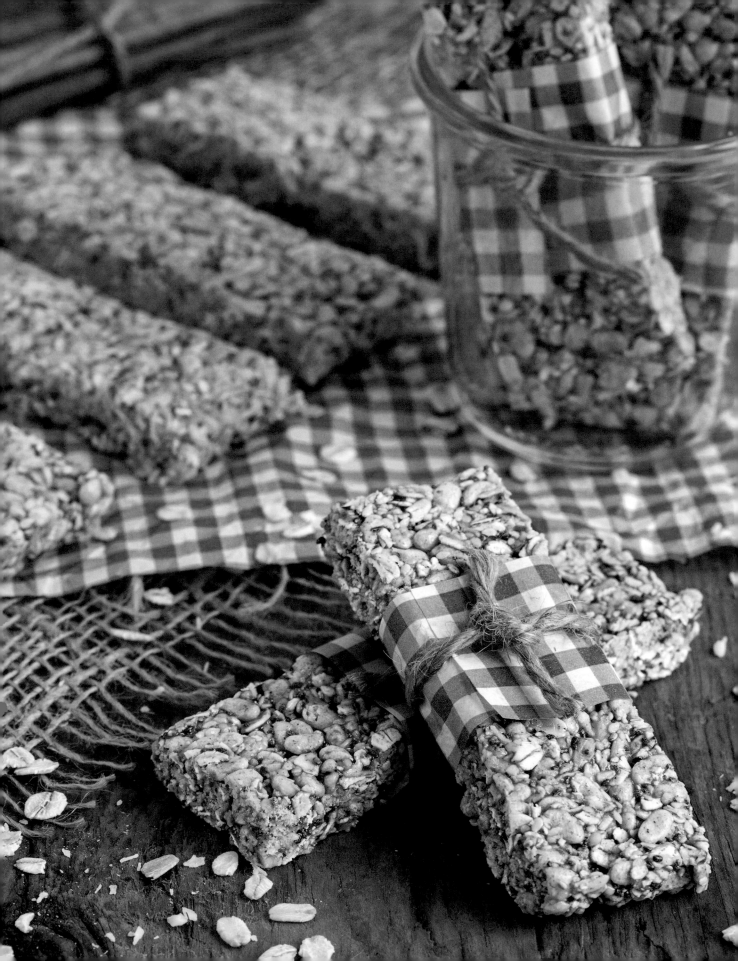

classic glo bar

150g gluten-free rolled oats

30g rice crisp cereal

35g hemp seeds

35g sunflower seeds

15g unsweetened shredded coconut

2 tablespoons sesame seeds

2 tablespoons chia seeds

½ teaspoon ground cinnamon

¼ teaspoon fine-grain sea salt

125ml plus 15ml brown rice syrup

60g roasted peanut butter or almond butter

1 teaspoon pure vanilla extract

45g mini non-dairy chocolate chips (such as Enjoy Life brand) (optional)

This is the granola bar that started it all! In 2009, I created a vegan energy bar recipe. To say it was an instant hit is an understatement. People online and offline went crazy for these bars, and they became so popular that I started getting all kinds of requests to sell my Glo Bars to adoring fans. Several months later, I opened an online vegan bakery featuring this Glo Bar and a handful of other flavours. I baked, by hand, more than five hundred Glo Bars each week. It was the adventure of a lifetime, and when I started writing this cookbook, I knew I wanted to feature a couple of the most popular Glo Bar recipes as a thank-you to my loyal customers. So here they are, dear Glo Bar fans – this is my thank-you for your incredible support over the years! And if you've never had a Glo Bar before, I hope you enjoy them just as much as we do!

Makes 12 bars

PREP TIME: 15 minutes • FREEZE TIME: 10 minutes
gluten-free, oil-free, raw/no-bake, soy-free,
refined sugar-free, nut-free option

1. Line a 2.5-litre square cake pan with two pieces of parchment paper (one going each way).

2. In a large bowl, combine the oats, rice crisp cereal, hemp seeds, sunflower seeds, coconut, sesame seeds, chia seeds, cinnamon, and salt and mix.

3. In a small saucepan, stir together the brown rice syrup and peanut butter until well combined. Cook over a medium to high heat until the mixture softens and bubbles slightly, then remove the pan from the heat and stir in the vanilla.

4. Pour the peanut butter mixture over the oat mixture, using a spatula to scrape every last bit out of the pan. Stir well with a large metal spoon until all of the oats and cereal are coated in the wet

mixture. (The resulting mixture will be very thick and difficult to stir. If you get tired, just picture me making five hundred of these bars in a row, and you'll feel better!) If using the chocolate chips, allow the mixture to cool slightly before folding in the chips. This will prevent them from melting.

5. Transfer the mixture to the prepared pan, spreading it out into an even layer. Lightly wet your hands and press down on the mixture to even it out. Use a pastry roller to compact the mixture firmly and evenly. This helps the bars hold together better. Press down on the edges with your fingers to even out the mixture.

6. Place the pan in the freezer, uncovered, and chill for 10 minutes, or until firm.

7. Lift the oat square out of the pan, using the parchment paper as handles, and place it on a cutting board. With a pizza roller (or a serrated knife), slice the square into 6 rows and then slice them in half to make 12 bars total.

8. Wrap the bars individually in plastic wrap or foil and store them in an airtight container in the refrigerator for up to 2 weeks. Alternatively, you can store them in the freezer for up to 1 month.

Tip: To make the bars nut-free, substitute sunflower seed butter for the peanut butter. Look for lightly sweetened sunflower seed butter, such as by Sunbutter, because unsweetened sunflower seed butter can have a bitter aftertaste.

present glo bar

60g pecans, finely chopped

150g gluten-free rolled oats

30g rice crisp cereal

30g pepita seeds

30g dried cranberries

1 teaspoon ground cinnamon

¼ teaspoon kosher salt

125ml brown rice syrup

60g roasted almond butter or peanut butter

1 teaspoon pure vanilla extract

The Present Glo Bar was one of the most popular granola bars sold in my bakery, so this recipe was an obvious choice to put in the book. Filled with cinnamon, dried cranberries, pepita seeds, and toasted pecans, this granola bar reminds me of the holiday season. Enjoy this as my gift to you! I love to make several batches of these bars around the holidays and gift them to family and friends.

Makes 12 bars

PREP TIME: 10 minutes • CHILL TIME: 10 minutes

gluten-free, oil-free, soy-free, refined sugar-free

1. Preheat the oven to 150°C (300°F). Line a 2.5-litre square cake pan with two pieces of parchment paper (one going each way).

2. Spread the pecans in an even layer on a rimmed baking sheet and toast them in the oven for 10 to 12 minutes, until lightly golden and fragrant. Set aside to cool.

3. In a large bowl, combine the oats, rice crisp cereal, pepita seeds, cranberries, cinnamon, and salt. Stir in the cooled toasted pecans.

4. In a small saucepan, stir together the brown rice syrup and almond butter until well combined. Cook over a medium to high heat until the mixture softens and bubbles slightly, then remove the pan from the heat and stir in the vanilla.

5. Pour the almond butter mixture over the oat mixture, using a spatula to scrape every last bit out of the pan. Stir well until all of the oats and cereal are coated in the wet mixture. (The resulting mixture will be very thick and difficult to stir.)

6. Transfer the mixture to the prepared pan, spreading it out into an even layer. Lightly wet your hands and press down on the mixture to even it out. Use a pastry roller to compact the mixture firmly and

evenly. This helps the bars hold together better. Press down on the edges with your fingers to even out the mixture.

7. Place the pan in the freezer, uncovered, and chill for 10 minutes, or until firm.

8. Lift the oat square out of the pan, using the parchment paper as handles, and place it on a cutting board. With a pizza roller (or a serrated knife), slice the square into 6 rows and then slice them in half to make 12 bars total.

9. Wrap the bars individually in plastic wrap or foil and store them in an airtight container in the refrigerator for up to 2 weeks. Alternatively, you can store them in the freezer for up to 1 month.

....

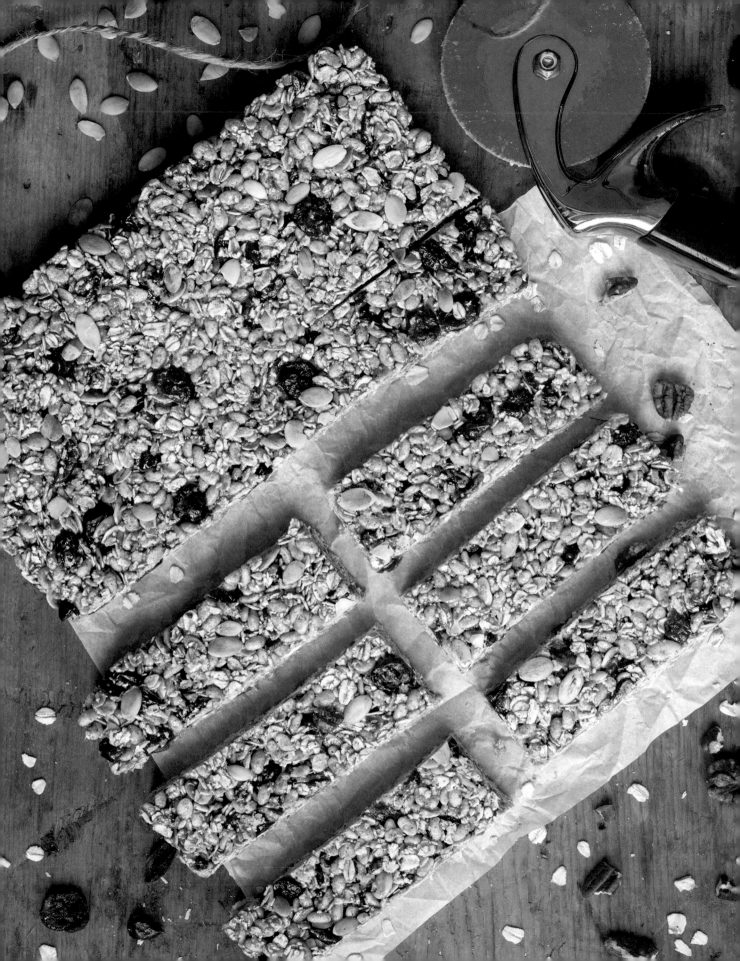

perfect roasted chickpeas

1 425g can chickpeas, drained and rinsed

½ teaspoon extra-virgin olive oil

1 teaspoon garlic powder

½ teaspoon fine-grain sea salt or Herbamare

½ teaspoon onion powder

¼ teaspoon cayenne pepper

Tip: If you have leftover roasted chickpeas, cool them completely and then store them in a container in the freezer for 5 to 7 days. To reheat, simply toss the frozen chickpeas on a baking sheet and roast them at 200°C (400°F) for 5 to 10 minutes, or until heated through. This restores the chickpeas to their former crunchy glory! Oh yeah.

This is my go-to all-purpose roasted chickpea recipe. After testing several different spice combinations, this was the one that everyone went crazy for. If you've never had roasted chickpeas before, you are in for a real treat! Once they are roasted, chickpeas become crunchy and chewy, which makes them the perfect pop-in-your-mouth high-protein snack. See my Tip below for storing and reheating leftover roasted chickpeas.

Serves 3

PREP TIME: 10 minutes • COOK TIME: 35 minutes

gluten-free, nut-free, soy-free, sugar-free, grain-free

1. Preheat the oven to 200°C (400°F). Line a large rimmed baking sheet with parchment paper.

2. Place a tea towel on the counter. Pour the chickpeas onto the tea towel and place another tea towel on top. Gently rub the chickpeas until completely dry. Carefully transfer the chickpeas to the prepared baking sheet.

3. Drizzle the chickpeas with the oil and roll them around until evenly coated.

4. Sprinkle the garlic powder, salt, onion powder, and cayenne over the chickpeas and roll them around until coated.

5. Roast the chickpeas for 20 minutes, and then shake the pan gently to roll the chickpeas around. Roast for 10 to 15 minutes more, until golden and lightly charred. Cool on the pan for 5 minutes and then serve.

salt & vinegar roasted chickpeas

1 425g can chickpeas, drained and rinsed

625ml white vinegar

1 teaspoon extra-virgin olive oil

½ teaspoon fine-grain sea salt or coarse sea salt, plus more as needed

Calling all salt and vinegar fans! This is my take on my favourite childhood snack – salt and vinegar crisps. To make this healthier version, simply boil chickpeas in vinegar, which infuses them with intense flavour. Then, you roast them with sea salt and a touch of olive oil until they are crunchy. As they say, once you pop, you can't stop. (But if you do, see the Tip on page 220 for storing leftover roasted chickpeas.)

Serves 3

PREP TIME: 30 minutes • COOK TIME: 30 to 35 minutes roasting

gluten-free, nut-free, soy-free, sugar-free, grain-free

1. Place the chickpeas and vinegar in a medium saucepan. Add a dash of sea salt. Bring the vinegar to a boil and cook for about 30 seconds, and then remove the pan from the heat. Some of the chickpea skins will fall off during this process, but not to worry. Cover the pan and let the chickpeas soak in the vinegar for 25 to 30 minutes.

2. Preheat the oven to 200°C (400°F). Line a large rimmed baking sheet with parchment paper.

3. Drain the chickpeas in a colander, discarding the vinegar. Shake off any excess vinegar, but there's no need to dry the chickpeas.

4. Transfer the chickpeas to the baking sheet and drizzle them with the oil. Massage the oil into the chickpeas with your fingers until fully coated. Sprinkle with the salt.

5. Roast the chickpeas for 20 minutes, and then give the pan a gentle shake to roll the chickpeas around on the pan. Roast for 10 to 15 minutes more, until golden and lightly charred.

6. Cool the chickpeas on the pan for 5 minutes. They will firm up as they cool.

Tip: I suggest turning on the range fan and opening a window when boiling the chickpeas in the vinegar, as the vinegar smell is very strong! As my husband says, it keeps away the vampires. Don't say I didn't warn you!

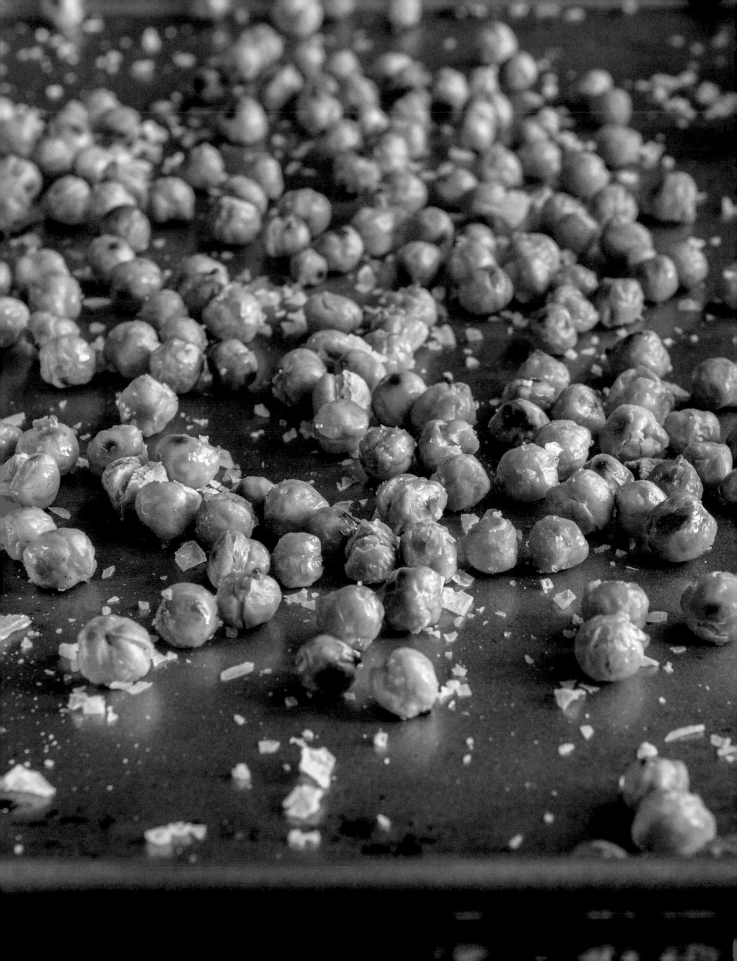

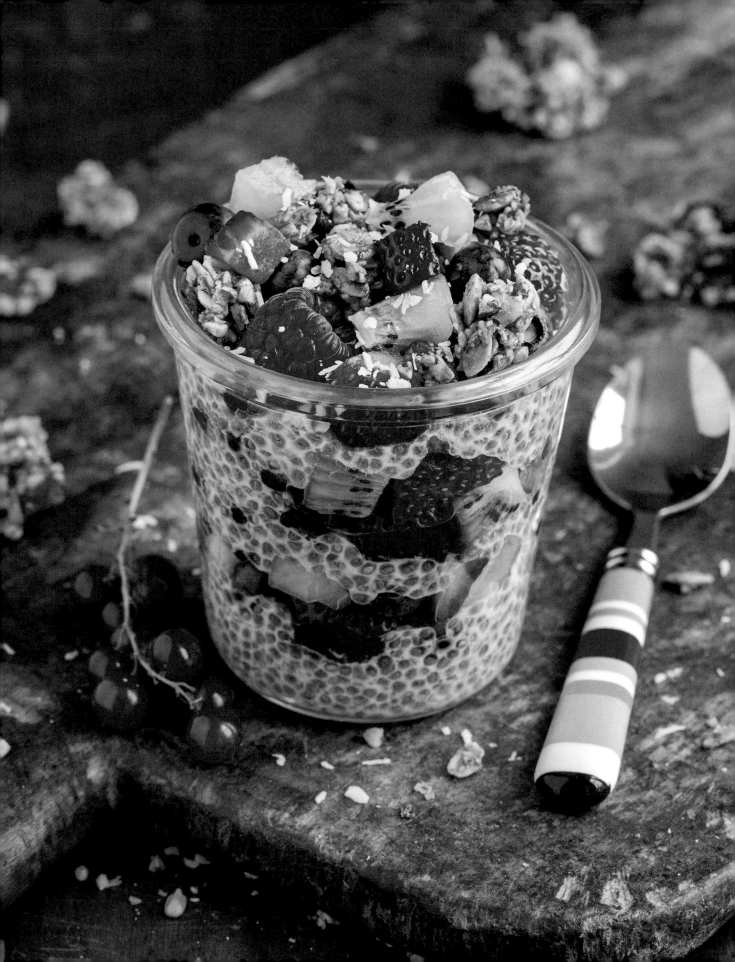

mighty chia pudding parfait

FOR THE PUDDING:

3 tablespoons chia seeds

250ml non-dairy milk

½ teaspoon pure vanilla extract

1½ to 3 teaspoons maple syrup or agave nectar, to taste

FOR LAYERING:

Fresh fruit

Ultimate Nutty Granola Clusters (see page 31)

Banana Soft Serve (see page 289) (optional)

Chia pudding is a tasty way to get a hefty dose of healthy omega-3 fatty acids, which give the skin a healthy glow. This pudding is especially creamy when it's made with my Creamy Vanilla Almond Milk (see page 275). The thickness of the chia pudding will vary based on the kind of milk you use, so don't worry if it looks a bit thick or thin when you first try it out. If your pudding is too thin, you can add more chia seeds and let it sit for thirty minutes more; if it's too thick, try adding a touch more almond milk. If you aren't a fan of the tapioca-like texture of chia seed pudding, whirl it in the blender before serving.

Serves 1

PREP TIME: 5 minutes • CHILL TIME: 8 hours or overnight

gluten-free, oil-free, raw/no-bake, soy-free, refined sugar-free, grain-free, nut-free option

1. In a medium bowl, whisk together the chia seeds, milk, vanilla, and maple syrup. Cover and refrigerate overnight, or for at least 2 hours, to thicken.

2. Serve the thickened, chilled pudding in parfait glasses, alternating it with layers of fresh fruit and granola. For a cool and creamy twist, layer Banana Soft Serve into the parfait as well.

Tip: For a nut-free option, use a nut-free non-dairy milk such as coconut milk.

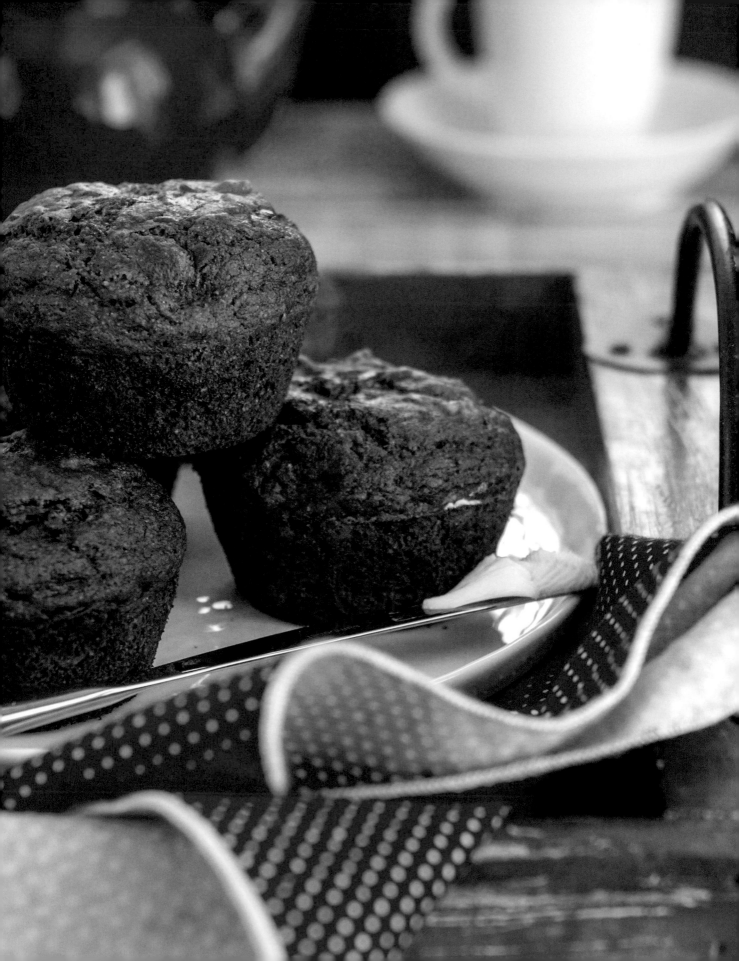

oil-free chocolate-courgette muffins

1 tablespoon ground flaxseed

300ml non-dairy milk

2 teaspoons apple cider vinegar or lemon juice

300g whole wheat pastry flour

110g Sucanat, coconut sugar, or natural cane sugar

40g unsweetened cocoa powder, sifted

1½ teaspoons baking powder

½ teaspoon baking soda

½ teaspoon fine-grain sea salt

3 tablespoons pure maple syrup

1 teaspoon pure vanilla extract

60g mini dark chocolate chips

85g walnuts, chopped (optional)

125g lightly packed grated courgette (about ½ medium courgette)

Lightly sweet and oil-free, these chocolate muffins are hiding a healthy green vegetable! Don't worry, you can't taste the courgette, but it does a fantastic job of adding moisture so we can do without any added oil. What's that? A vegan, refined sugar-free, and oil-free chocolate muffin that tastes great? Yes, it's true. Miracles do happen!

Makes 12 muffins
PREP TIME: 20 to 30 minutes
COOK TIME: 15 to 17 minutes
oil-free, soy-free, refined sugar-free, nut-free option

1. Preheat the oven to 180°C (350°F). Lightly grease a muffin tin with oil.

2. In a small bowl, stir together the ground flaxseed and 3 tablespoons of water. Set aside.

3. In a medium bowl, combine the milk and vinegar. Set aside. It will curdle a bit, but that's the point – we're making vegan buttermilk.

4. In a large bowl, combine the flour, sugar, cocoa powder, baking powder, baking soda, and salt.

5. To the bowl with the milk and vinegar mixture, stir in the flaxseed mixture, the maple syrup, and the vanilla. Pour the milk mixture over the flour mixture and stir until just combined. Fold in the chocolate chips, walnuts (if using), and courgette, being careful not to over-mix.

6. Spoon the batter into the prepared muffin tin, filling each well three-quarters full. Bake for 15 to 17 minutes, or until the muffins slowly spring back when touched. A toothpick inserted into the

centre of a muffin should come out clean. Cool the muffins in the tin for 5 minutes.

7. Run a knife around the edges of the muffins to release them from the pan and transfer them to a rack to cool completely.

Tip : For a nut-free option, omit the walnuts.

super-power chia bread

50g gluten-free rolled oats

25g raw buckwheat groats (or more rolled oats)

80g chia seeds

35g raw sunflower seeds

30g raw pepita seeds

1 teaspoon dried oregano

1 teaspoon sugar (optional)

½ teaspoon dried thyme

½ teaspoon fine-grain sea salt, plus more as needed

¼ teaspoon garlic powder

¼ teaspoon onion powder

Chewy, hearty, and dense – this isn't your average slice of bread! Packed with 9 grams of protein and more than 7 grams of fibre per slice, this bread will keep you going for hours and is a healthier alternative to store-bought bread. Since it's a staple in our kitchen, I make a double batch every week. Feel free to play around with the herbs and spices as you see fit!

Serves 8

PREP TIME: 5 minutes   •   BAKE TIME: 30 minutes

gluten-free, nut-free, oil-free, soy-free, sugar-free option

1. Preheat the oven to 160°C (325°F). Line a 2.5-litre square cake pan with two pieces of parchment paper, one going each way.

2. Place the oats and buckwheat groats in a high-speed blender and blend on the highest speed until a fine flour forms.

3. In a large bowl, combine the oat and buckwheat flour, chia seeds, sunflower seeds, pepita seeds, oregano, sugar (if using), thyme, salt, garlic powder, and onion powder and stir until well combined.

4. Stir in 250ml water until combined. The mixture will be very watery and runny.

5. Pour the mixture into the pan and spread it out evenly with a spatula. You can use lightly wet hands to smooth it level, if necessary. Sprinkle the surface with some additional salt.

6. Bake, uncovered, for about 25 minutes, or until firm to the touch. Let the bread cool in the pan for 5 minutes and then transfer it to a cooling rack to cool for 5 to 10 minutes more. Slice and enjoy!

Tips: This bread keeps in an airtight container in the fridge for 2 to 3 days – any longer and it starts to get a gummy texture. I prefer to freeze leftover bread and simply thaw it in the fridge before I use it.

I love toasting this bread and then spreading it with coconut oil, nut butter, or hummus. Try it for yourself!

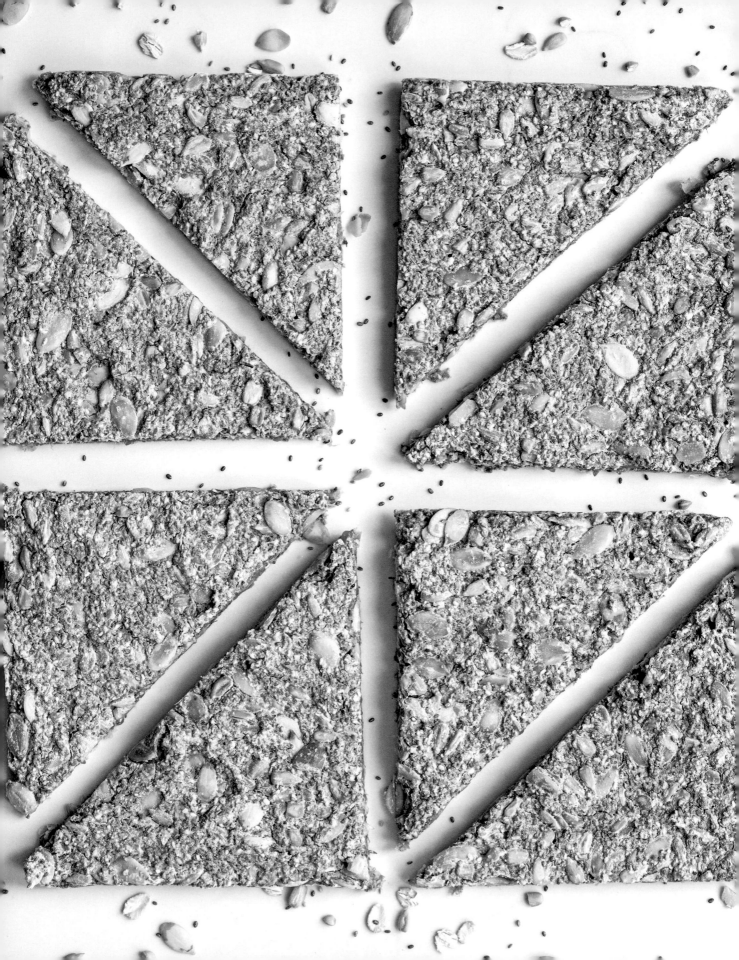

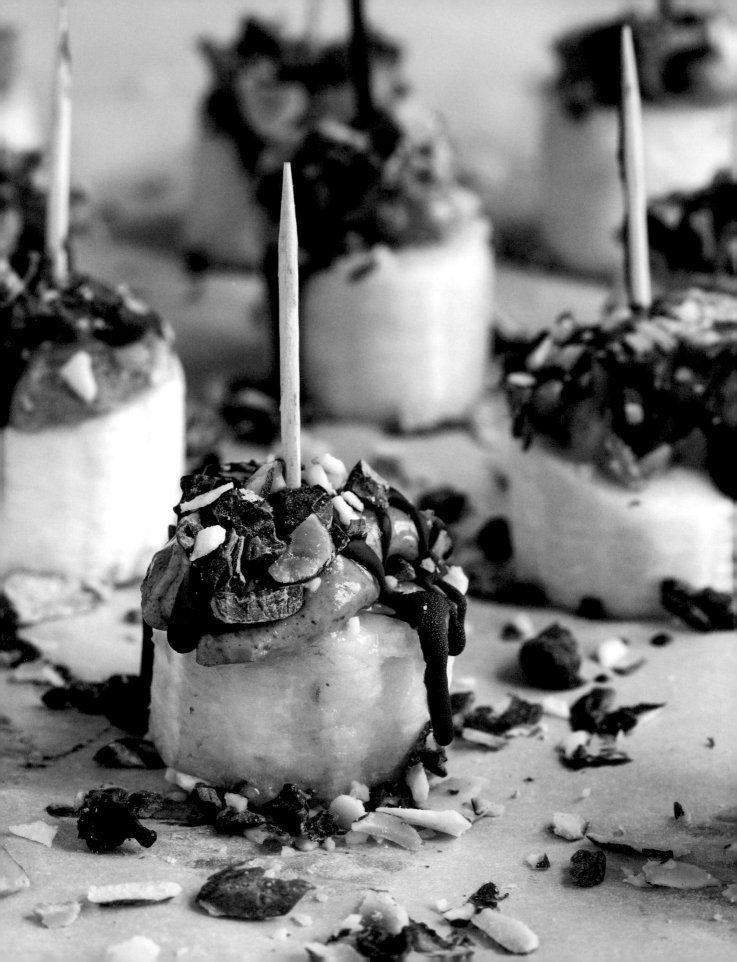

cacao crunch almond butter-banana bites

2 large bananas, peeled and sliced crosswise into 2cm-wide pieces

3 tablespoons roasted chunky almond butter or peanut butter

2 tablespoons dark chocolate chips

½ teaspoon coconut oil

1 tablespoon raw cacao nibs

2 teaspoons toasted sliced almonds

Meet my healthier solution to a loaded ice cream sundae. Frozen banana bites mimic the creamy texture of ice cream, while the crunchy toppings make it a party in your mouth! I strongly recommend using crunchy roasted nut butter if you can get your hands on some (or try my Crunchy Maple-Cinnamon Roasted Almond Butter, page 295). The nut pieces give this snack a great texture and the roasted flavour can't be beaten.

Makes 18 bites

PREP TIME: 10 minutes • FREEZE TIME: 30 to 40 minutes

gluten-free, raw/no-bake, grain-free

1. Line a large plate with a piece of parchment paper. Place the sliced bananas on the parchment paper. Carefully spread ½ teaspoon of the almond butter on top of each banana piece.

2. Place the plate in the freezer to chill for at least 30 minutes, until the banana firms up.

3. In a small saucepan, gently melt the chocolate chips and oil together over a very low heat. Stir to combine. With a small spoon, drizzle some of the melted chocolate on top of each banana piece.

4. Immediately sprinkle the banana pieces with the cacao nibs and almond slices and stick a toothpick in each (if desired). The melted chocolate will quickly harden up. If this doesn't happen, simply place the plate back in the freezer for 5 to 10 minutes more, until the chocolate hardens.

5. Serve immediately. Store leftovers in a container in the freezer. Partially thaw on the counter for a few minutes, before serving.

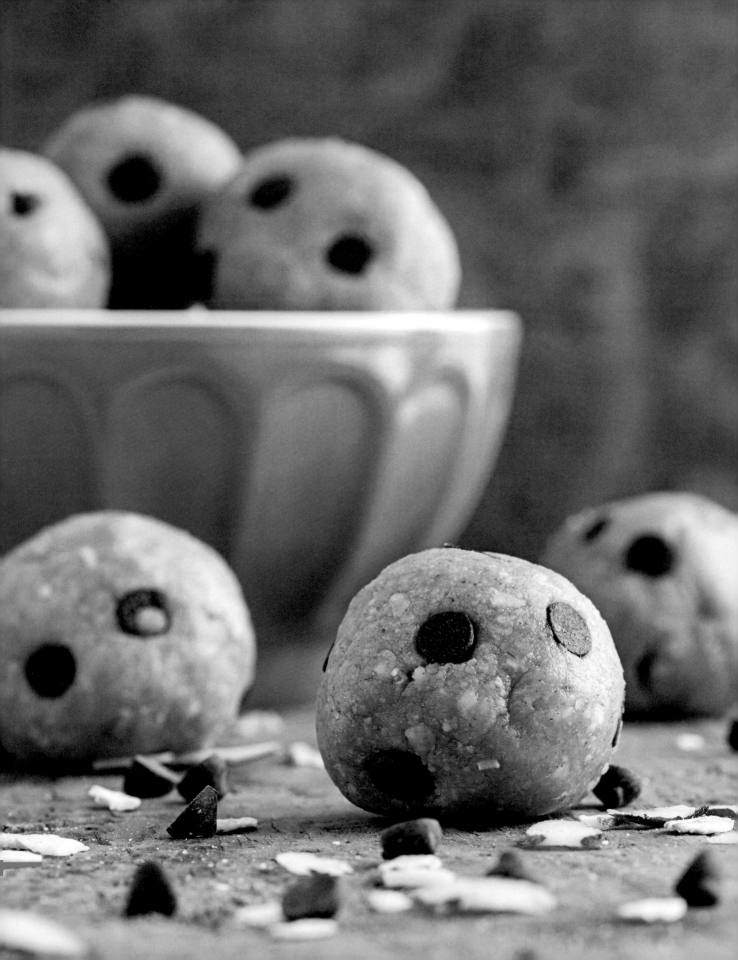

peanut butter cookie dough bites

150g gluten-free rolled oats

2 tablespoons coconut oil

2 tablespoons smooth peanut butter, almond butter, or sunflower seed butter

60ml pure maple syrup or other liquid sweetener

1 teaspoon pure vanilla extract

60g almond flour or almond meal

¼ teaspoon fine-grain sea salt

2 tablespoons mini dark chocolate chips or chopped dark chocolate

Tips: For a nut-free version, simply swap sunflower seed butter for the peanut butter and more oat flour for the almond flour (add a splash of non-dairy milk if the dough is a bit dry). Both versions work just fine.

For a soy-free option, use soy-free chocolate chips (such as Enjoy Life brand)

When I was growing up, my best friend, Allison, and I used to split an entire package of store-bought cookie dough for a snack. Yes, as a *snack*! We'd slice the plastic cookie dough package down the middle, grab two spoons, and go to town eating the raw dough. Oh, to be kids again! I'm happy to say that my love for cookie dough has never dwindled, but I now make my own using all-natural ingredients. My health, arteries, and waistline thank me. Best of all, these cookie dough bites are still very much kid-approved.

Makes 14 small bites
PREP TIME: 15 minutes • CHILL TIME: 10 minutes
gluten-free, raw/no-bake, soy-free option,
nut-free option, refined sugar-free

1. In a high-speed blender, blend the oats until a fine flour forms. Set aside.

2. In a large bowl, combine the oil, peanut butter, maple syrup, and vanilla and beat with a hand mixer until smooth. Add the almond flour, oat flour, and salt and beat again until combined. Fold in the chocolate chips.

3. Roll the dough into small balls (about 1 tablespoon of dough each). If chocolate chips fall to the bottom of the bowl, press them back into the dough when rolling. Place the finished bites on a plate lined with parchment paper.

4. Freeze the bites for 5 to 10 minutes, or until firm. Store the bites in the freezer in a freezer bag for quick and easy snacks.

desserts

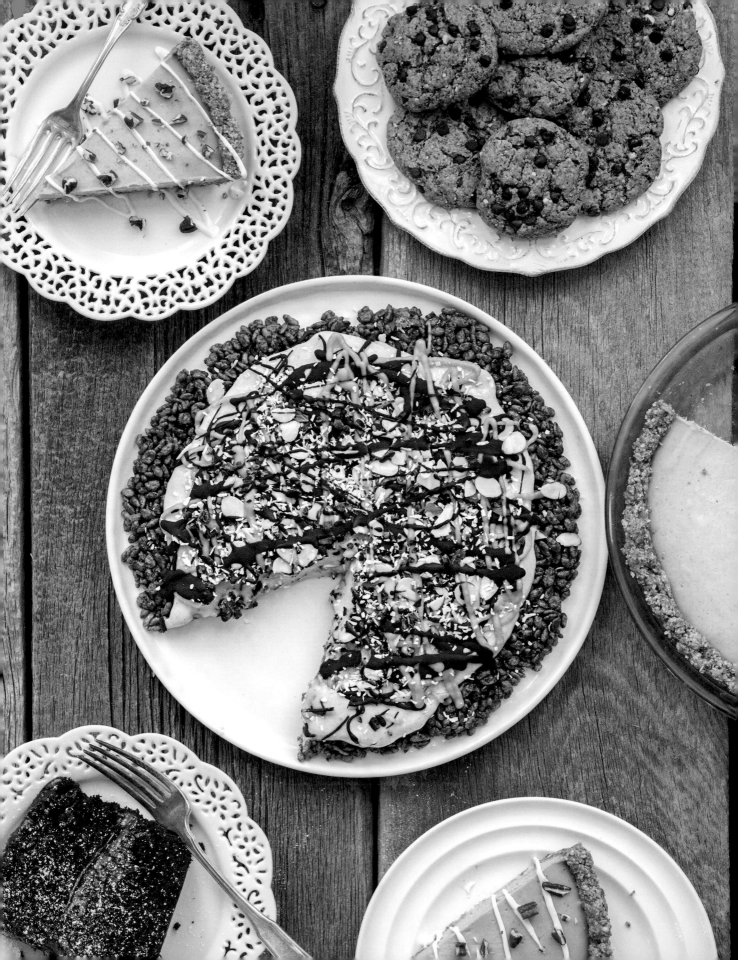

I've always had the sweet tooth in my family. Since I was a little girl, I've preferred sweets over salty snacks, and even today it's rare when I don't end my day with something sweet. It could be as simple as a couple of squares of dark chocolate or fresh fruit, or if we're entertaining I'll often pull out all the stops with a decadent dessert like my Chilled Chocolate-Espresso Torte with Toasted Hazelnut Crust (page 241) or my Double-Layer Chocolate Fudge Cake (page 249). Life is just too short not to enjoy dessert. The best part about my desserts – aside from how mouthwatering they are – is that they are made with wholesome ingredients. I prefer to use whole grain flours like oat flour, almond flour, or whole wheat pastry flour and natural sweeteners like maple syrup, coconut sugar, or Medjool dates whenever possible. It really does make a difference to how you feel when you indulge. If you are looking for a quick fix for your sweet tooth, try one of my no-bake desserts like Homemade Yolos (page 263) or Beat the Heat Frozen Dessert Pizza (page 269). Crispy Almond Butter Chocolate Chip Cookies (page 265) are also quick to throw together and are perfect served with a cold glass of Creamy Vanilla Almond Milk (see page 275). I'm drooling just thinking about it.

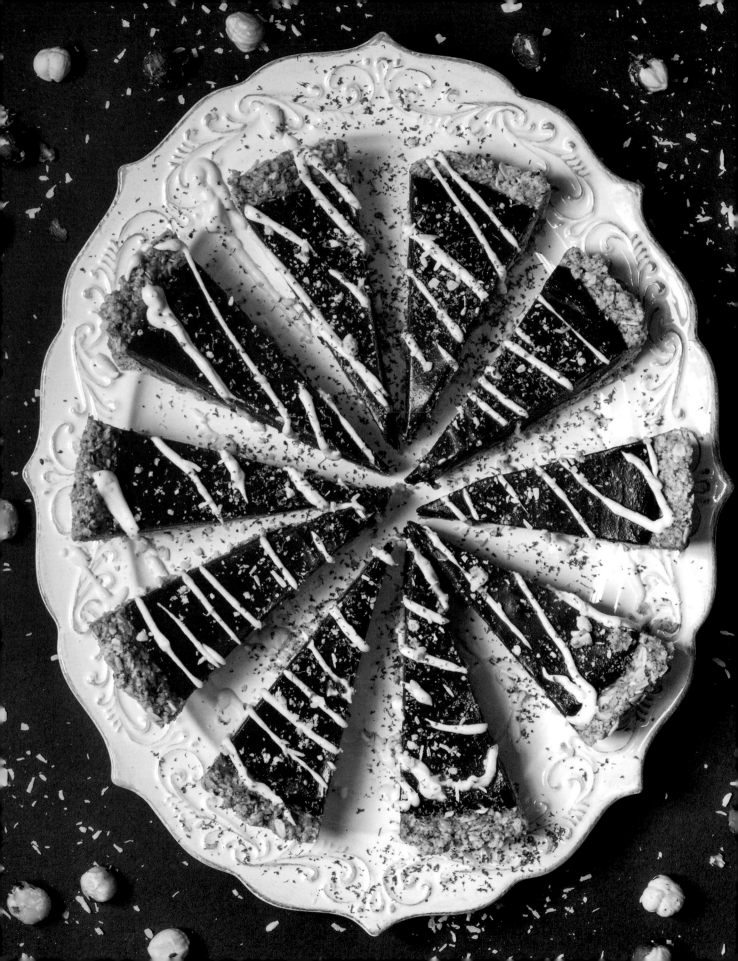

chilled chocolate-espresso torte with toasted hazelnut crust

FOR THE TOASTED HAZELNUT CRUST:

75g raw hazelnuts

60ml coconut oil

3 tablespoons maple syrup

¼ teaspoon fine-grain sea salt

50g gluten-free oat flour

100g gluten-free rolled oats

FOR THE CHOCOLATE FILLING:

225g cashews, soaked
(see page 11)

150ml agave nectar, or 175ml pure maple syrup

125ml coconut oil

35g cocoa powder

60g dark chocolate chips, melted

2 teaspoons pure vanilla extract

½ teaspoon fine-grain sea salt

½ teaspoon espresso powder (optional)

Shaved chocolate (optional)

Coconut flakes (optional)

This is a crowd-pleasing chocolate dessert that will win over any chocolate fan. Reminiscent of Nutella, the popular chocolate-hazelnut spread, my toasted hazelnut crust is the perfect nutty complement to the rich and creamy chocolate filling. No one will believe this torte is dairy-free and many will go back for seconds despite their best intentions. If you want a show-stopping dessert that will wow a crowd, this is your recipe. Be sure to soak the cashews overnight, or for at least three to four hours, so they're ready when you need them.

Makes 1 23cm torte; serves 8 to 14
PREP TIME: 30 to 35 minutes
FREEZE TIME: 4 to 6 hours minimum, but preferably overnight
gluten-free

1. Make the Toasted Hazelnut Crust: Preheat the oven to 180°C (350°F). Lightly grease a 23cm pie dish with coconut oil.

2. In a food processor, process the hazelnuts into a fine crumb with the texture of sand. Add the oil, maple syrup, salt, and oat flour and process again until the dough comes together. Finally, add the rolled oats and pulse until the oats are chopped but still have some texture to them. The dough should stick together slightly when pressed between your fingers, but it shouldn't be super-sticky either. If it's too dry, try adding 1 teaspoon of water or processing a bit longer.

3. With your fingers, crumble the dough evenly over the base of the pie dish. Starting from the middle, press the mixture firmly and evenly into the dish, moving outward and upward along the side of the pie dish. The harder you press the crumbs into the dish, the better the crust will hold together. Poke a few fork holes into the bottom to let steam escape.

4. Bake the crust, uncovered, for 10 to 13 minutes, until lightly golden. Remove from the oven and set aside to cool on a rack for 15 to 20 minutes.

5. Make the Filling: Drain and rinse the cashews. In a high-speed blender, combine the soaked cashews, agave, oil, cocoa powder, melted chocolate, vanilla, salt, and espresso powder (if using) and blend on high until the filling is completely smooth. It can take a few minutes of blending to get it smooth, depending on your blender. If the blender needs more liquid to get it going, add a tablespoon of almond milk (or a bit more) to help it along.

6. Pour the filling into the prepared crust, scooping every last bit out of the blender. Smooth out the top evenly. Garnish with shaved chocolate and/or coconut flakes, if desired.

7. Place the pie dish on an even surface in the freezer, uncovered. Freeze for a couple of hours, and then cover the dish with foil and freeze overnight, or for a minimum of 4 to 6 hours, until the pie sets.

8. Remove the pie from the freezer and let it sit on the counter for 10 minutes before slicing. **This pie is meant to be served frozen.** Serve with homemade Whipped Coconut Cream (see page 280) and finely chopped hazelnuts, if desired, but it's fantastic all on its own, too. Wrap leftover slices individually in foil and store them in an airtight container in the freezer for 1 to 1½ weeks.

Tip: Not in the mood to make a crust? Turn this dessert into freezer fudge by preparing only the chocolate filling. Pour the filling into a 20cm square pan lined with plastic wrap; top with 60g toasted hazelnuts or walnuts, and freeze until solid (about 2 hours). Slice into squares and enjoy straight from the freezer.

mother nature's apple crumble

FOR THE APPLE FILLING:

6 to 7 baking apples, peeled and chopped (see Tip, page 244)

1 tablespoon arrowroot powder or cornstarch

225g Sucanat sugar or other granulated sugar

1 tablespoon chia seeds (optional)

1 teaspoon ground cinnamon

1 tablespoon fresh lemon juice

FOR THE TOPPING:

100g gluten-free rolled oats

110g thinly sliced almonds

40g almond flour or almond meal

60ml pure maple syrup

60ml coconut oil, melted

2 tablespoons unsweetened shredded coconut (optional)

1 teaspoon ground cinnamon

¼ teaspoon fine-grain sea salt

Bid farewell to traditional apple crisps, many of which are loaded with white sugar, bleached white flour, and butter. This flour- and refined sugar-free version is about as wholesome as it gets, and it still pleases kids and adults alike. Serve it with a scoop of your favourite vegan ice cream or Whipped Coconut Cream (see page 280) to take it over the top. If you want to change it up, try using a mix of apples and pears for a fun twist.

Makes 8 small servings
PREP TIME: 25 to 30 minutes
COOK TIME: 45 to 60 minutes
gluten-free, soy-free, refined sugar-free

1. Preheat the oven to 190°C (375°F). Lightly grease a 2.5-litre baking dish.

2. Make the Apple Filling: Place the apples in a large bowl and sprinkle the arrowroot powder on top. Toss until combined. Stir in the sugar, chia seeds, and cinnamon. Add the lemon juice and stir to combine. Pour the apple mixture into the prepared dish and smooth it out evenly.

3. Make the Topping: In a large bowl (you can use the same one you used for the apples), stir together the oats, almonds, almond flour, maple syrup, melted coconut oil, shredded coconut (if using), cinnamon, and salt until thoroughly mixed.

4. Sprinkle the oat mixture all over the apple mixture in an even layer.

5. Cover the dish with foil and poke a couple of air holes in the foil. Bake for 35 to 45 minutes, until the apples are just fork-tender. Uncover the dish and bake for 10 to 15 minutes more, until the topping is golden and fragrant.

6. Serve with a scoop of dairy-free vanilla ice cream or Whipped Coconut Cream (see page 280). The leftovers are fantastic cold, straight from the fridge, or you can reheat it in the oven for 15 to 20 minutes. It's healthy enough for breakfast the next day, too!

Tip: I like to use a variety of apples for the best flavour. I often use a mix of Honeycrisp, Granny Smith, and Gala apples with great results. This crumble works with other fruit, too, so use whatever is in season. Peaches and blueberries are a nice combo, although they produce a much juicer (and occasionally watery) crumble.

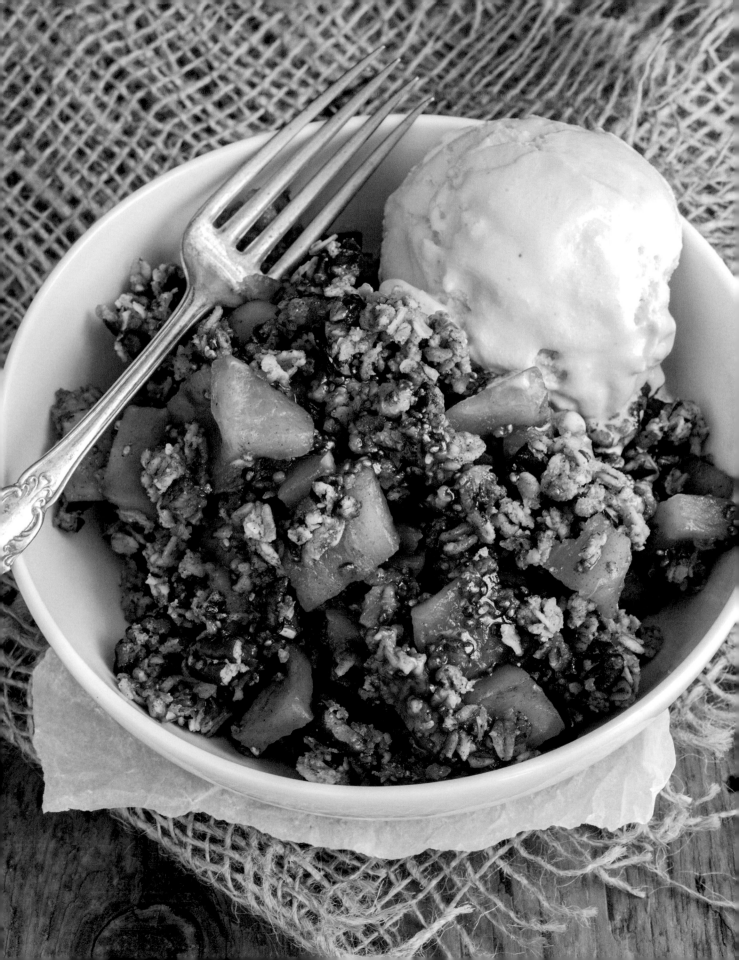

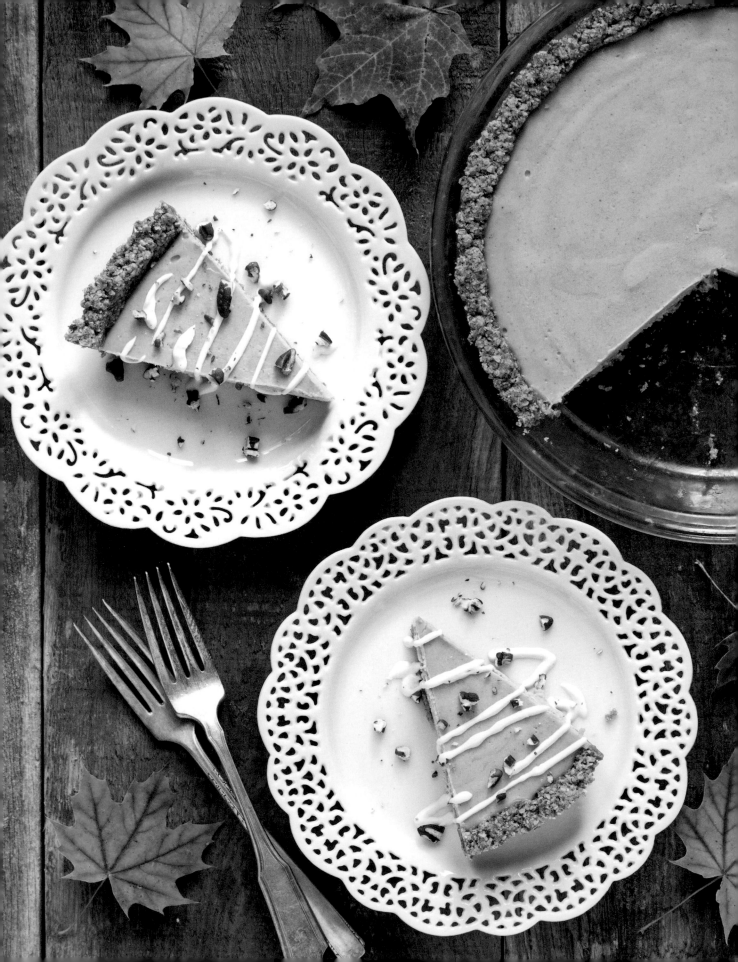

raw pumpkin-maple pie with baked oat crust

FOR THE CRUST:

140g pitted Medjool dates

125g gluten-free rolled oats

50g pecans

¼ teaspoon ground cinnamon

⅛ teaspoon salt

3 tablespoons coconut oil, at room temperature

FOR THE FILLING:

150g raw cashews, soaked (see page 11)

225g canned pumpkin purée

175ml pure maple syrup

125ml coconut oil

2 teaspoons pure vanilla extract

¾ teaspoon ground cinnamon

¼ teaspoon fine-grain sea salt

⅛ teaspoon ground ginger

⅛ teaspoon freshly grated or pre-ground nutmeg

FOR SERVING:

Whipped Coconut Cream (see page 280) (optional)

Finely chopped pecans (optional)

Freshly grated nutmeg (optional)

I brought this pumpkin pie to a recent holiday dinner (along with my Chilled Chocolate-Espresso Torte – see page 241) and everyone raved about it – even the pumpkin haters in the group! There wasn't a crumb left on anyone's plate and I was grinning from ear to ear. The no-bake filling is rich and decadent thanks to the creamy cashew base, so I like to serve it in small slivers – a little bit goes a long way. Be sure to serve this pie chilled; just a five- to ten-minute thaw on the counter is all that stands between you and your guests enjoying dessert. It also needs to set overnight in the freezer, so be sure to prep this the day before you need it. Soak the cashews overnight, or for at least three to four hours, so they're ready to go when you need them.

Makes 1 23cm torte; serves 8 to 14

PREP TIME: 25 minutes • FREEZE TIME: 5 hours minimum
gluten-free, soy-free, refined sugar free

1. Make the Crust: Preheat the oven to 180°C (350°F). Lightly grease a 23cm pie dish with coconut oil. If your dates are firm, soak them in water for 30 to 60 minutes and drain before using.

2. In a food processor, combine the oats, pecans, cinnamon, and salt and process until the mixture has the texture of coarse sand. Add the dates and oil and process again until the mixture comes together. It should stick together when pressed with your fingers. If it's dry, add 1 teaspoon of water and process again.

3. Sprinkle the crust mixture all over the base of the pie dish. Starting from the middle, press the crumbs firmly and evenly into the dish in an outward direction. The harder you press the crumbs into the dish, the more it will hold together. Push the crust up along the sides of the dish and even out the edge with your fingers. Poke

several fork holes in the crust and bake, uncovered, for 10 to 12 minutes, until lightly golden. Set aside to cool for 30 minutes on a cooling rack.

4. Make the Filling: Drain and rinse the cashews. In a high-speed blender, combine the soaked cashews, pumpkin, maple syrup, oil, vanilla, cinnamon, salt, ginger, and nutmeg and blend on high until completely smooth. This can take a few minutes, depending on your blender. If your blender needs more liquid to get it going, add 1 tablespoon of almond milk (or a bit more) to help it along.

5. Pour the filling into the semi-cooled crust and smooth out the top. Carefully cover the dish with foil and place on an even surface in the freezer to chill overnight, or for at least 5 to 6 hours, until firm.

6. Remove the pie from the freezer and let it sit on the counter for 10 minutes before slicing. This pie is meant to be served cold, and it tastes best served frozen. Serve with homemade Whipped Coconut Cream, finely chopped pecans, and freshly grated nutmeg, if desired.

Tips: Leftover pie will keep in the freezer for up to 10 days. Wrap each slice individually in plastic wrap or tin foil and store them in an airtight container.

Not in the mood to make a crust? Turn this dessert into freezer fudge by preparing only the pumpkin filling. Pour the filling into a 20cm square pan lined with plastic wrap, top with 60g toasted pecans, and freeze until solid (1½ to 2 hours). Slice into squares and enjoy straight from the freezer!

double-layer chocolate fudge cake

500ml non-dairy milk

2 tablespoons apple cider vinegar or white vinegar

340g natural cane sugar (see Tips, page 250)

150ml melted coconut oil or grapeseed oil

2 tablespoons pure vanilla extract (yes, that's correct!)

150g whole wheat pastry flour

200g all-purpose flour

65g cocoa powder, sifted

2 teaspoons baking soda

1¼ teaspoons fine-grain sea salt

1 recipe Chocolate Buttercream or Chocolate-Avocado Frosting (see page 288)

Shaved dark chocolate (optional)

Everyone needs a go-to double-layer chocolate cake in their baking holster for special occasions, and this chocolaty delight is the cake I make most often for birthdays and other special events. It's always a hit with kids and adults alike and it's a great dessert to show the sceptics that vegan desserts can taste even better than traditional desserts! In fact, my mom says this is the best chocolate cake she has ever made, vegan or otherwise. Aren't moms the best? I snuck in whole wheat pastry flour to boost the nutrition and also used unbleached organic all-purpose flour and natural cane sugar, instead of the bleached stuff. If you aren't in the mood for a double-layer cake, see my Tips on page 250 for turning this cake into cupcakes or a rectangular sheet cake. I've got you covered.

Serves 14

PREP TIME: 30 minutes • COOK TIME: 30 to 35 minutes

nut-free, soy-free, refined sugar-free

1. Preheat the oven to 180°C (350°F). Lightly grease two 1-litre cake pans and line the base with a circle of parchment paper. If making cupcakes, line a cupcake tin with paper liners.

2. In a medium bowl, stir together the milk and vinegar. Set it aside for a minute or two. This combination makes vegan buttermilk.

3. Add the sugar, oil, and vanilla to the bowl with the milk. Whisk to combine.

4. In a large bowl, whisk together the pastry flour, all-purpose flour, cocoa powder, baking soda, and salt until combined.

5. Pour the milk mixture over the flour mixture and beat with a hand mixer until smooth.

6. Divide the batter evenly between the prepared cake pans and smooth out the tops.

7. Bake the cakes for 30 to 35 minutes, rotating the pans halfway through the baking time. The cake is ready when it slowly springs back when touched and a toothpick inserted in the centre comes out clean. Place the pans on a cooling rack to cool for 20 to 25 minutes. Now slide a butter knife around the cake to loosen the edge. Gently and carefully invert the cakes onto a cooling rack. Let cool for 30 to 45 minutes more.

8. Once the cakes are completely cool, place a piece of parchment paper on top of a cake stand. Place one layer of the cake in the center of the parchment paper. With a serrated knife, trim the bottom layer until it's flat and level, if desired. Spread a layer of frosting on top. Place the second layer on top and gently push down to adhere.

9. Continue frosting the rest of the cake, starting at the top and then moving around to the sides. Garnish the frosted cake with shaved chocolate, if desired. Remove parchment from underneath cake. Leftover cake will stay fresh wrapped in plastic wrap or tin foil at room temperature for 3 to 4 days.

Tips: If you don't want to make this as a double-layer cake, rest assured that it can be made into cupcakes or a rectangular cake as well. The batter makes enough for 24 cupcakes. Bake the cupcakes for 21 to 25 minutes, or until a toothpick comes out clean and the cupcakes spring back slowly when touched. Allow the cupcakes to cool completely before frosting. You can also make this into one rectangular sheet cake. Pour the batter into a greased 23 by 33cm rectangular cake pan and bake for 31 to 35 minutes, or until a toothpick comes out clean and the cake springs back slowly when touched. Cool the cake completely and then frost as above.

I do not recommend subbing another type of sugar such as coconut or Sucanat sugar for the natural cane sugar. These sugars tend to dry out and crack the top of the cake when used. For best results, always use natural cane sugar in this cake recipe.

Last, keep in mind that 100% whole wheat flour should *not* be used as a substitute for whole wheat pastry flour, as it produces a dense, heavy cake.

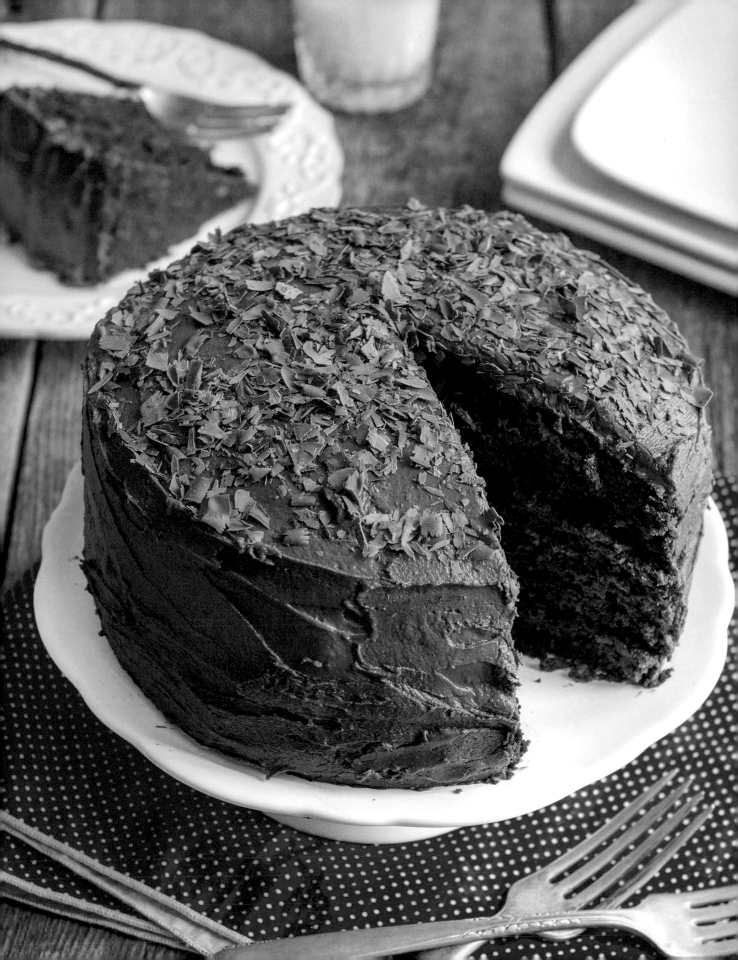

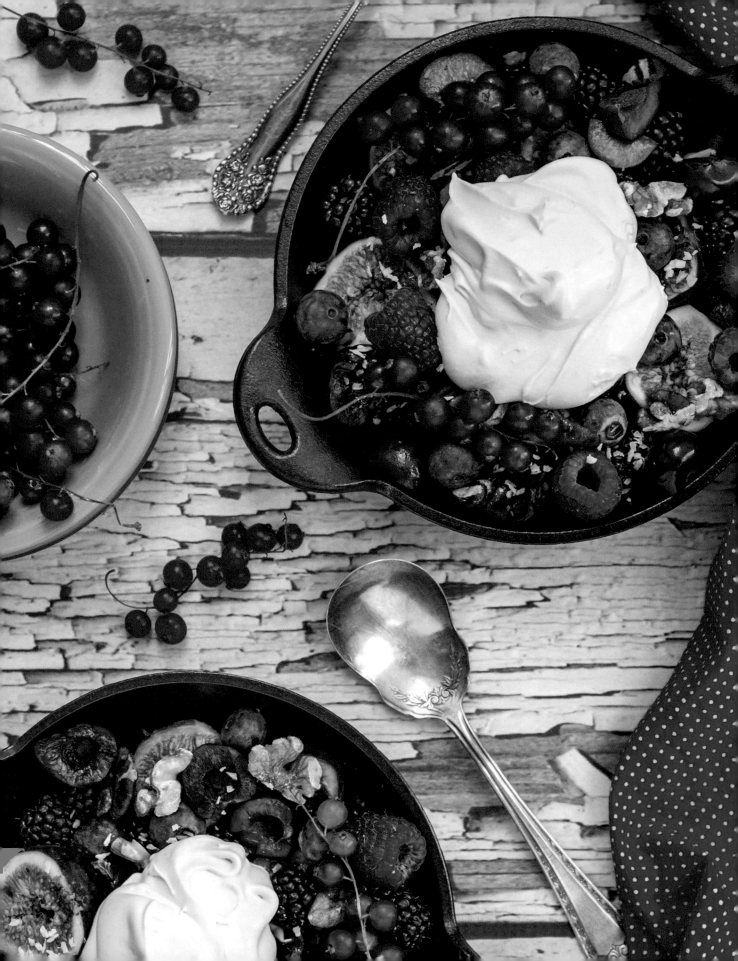

fresh fruit, nuts & whipped coconut cream

175g mixed nuts, roughly chopped

700g mixed in-season fresh fruit

1 recipe Whipped Coconut Cream (see page 280)

Sometimes the simplest desserts are the best. This is an effortless summer dessert that my husband and I enjoy whenever we have a bowl of fresh fruit to use up. Simply place some seasonal fruit in a bowl, top it with toasted nuts, and add a dollop of Whipped Coconut Cream on top. It doesn't get much easier than this, but it still looks fancy enough to serve to guests. Add a shaving of dark chocolate on top for the chocolate lovers.

Serves 6

PREP TIME: 20 minutes

gluten-free, oil-free, soy-free, refined sugar-free, grain-free

1. Preheat the oven to 150°C (300°F). Spread the nuts in a single layer on a rimmed baking sheet and toast them in the oven for 8 to 12 minutes, until lightly golden and fragrant.

2. Place a generous portion of fresh fruit in a small bowl or parfait glass. Add some Whipped Coconut Cream and top with a sprinkle of toasted nuts.

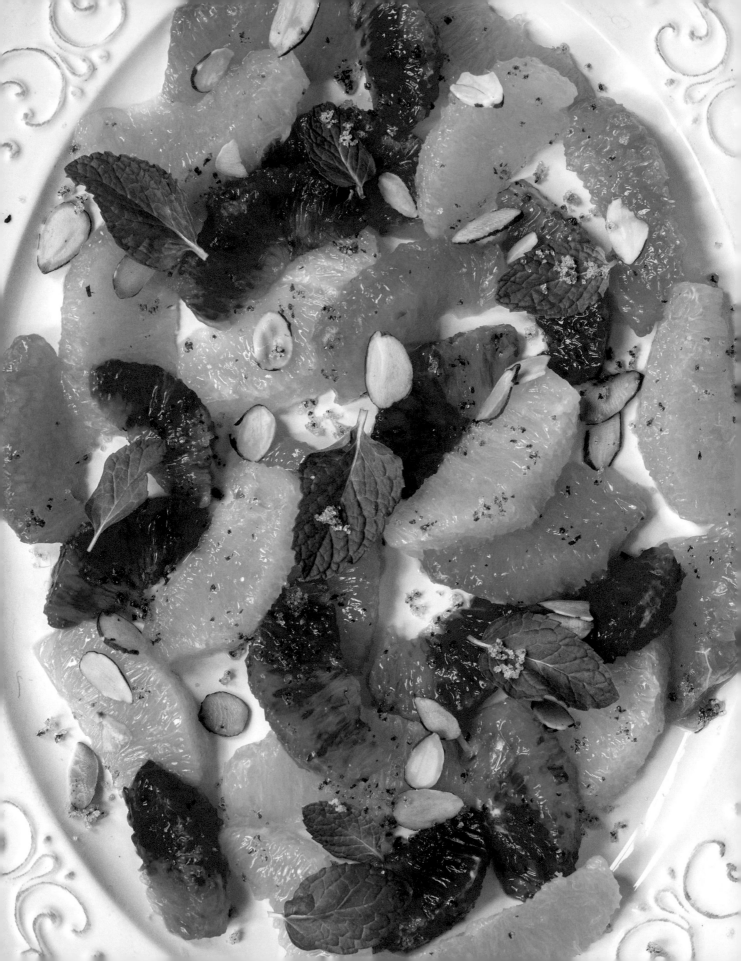

winter citrus salad

1 red grapefruit

2 navel oranges

2 blood oranges

2 tablespoons natural cane sugar

2 tablespoons fresh mint leaves, plus more for serving

2 tablespoons toasted almond slices, for serving (optional)

This is one of my favourite winter treats – in-season citrus accented with an energizing mint sugar garnish and toasted almonds. The process of segmenting citrus fruit is a bit tedious, but it's well worth the effort to make this light, gorgeous, and energizing cold-weather dessert. When you're struggling through the dreary days of winter, make this salad for a dose of sunshine in your life.

Serves 2

PREP TIME: 20 to 30 minutes

gluten-free, nut-free option, oil-free, raw/no-bake, soy-free, grain-free, refined sugar-free

1. Segment the grapefruit and oranges: Slice 1 to 2cm off the top and bottom off the citrus fruit so the inner flesh is exposed. With a paring knife, slice the skin and white pith off the fruit. Now cut out the segments in between the membranes. Place the segments on a plate and repeat for the rest of the citrus.

2. In a food processor, process the sugar and mint leaves together until finely chopped. The sugar should look green. Sprinkle the mint sugar over the citrus segments. Top with fresh mint leaves and toasted almond slices, if desired.

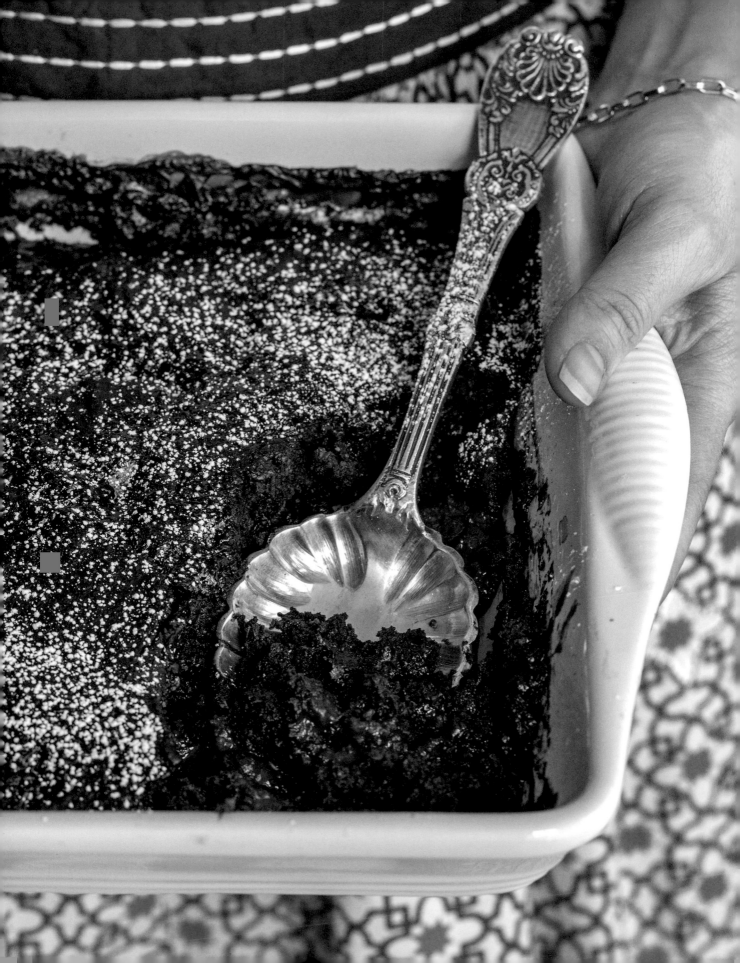

fudgy mocha pudding cake

1 tablespoon ground flaxseed

150g gluten-free oat flour

170g plus 75g coconut sugar or other granulated sugar

35g plus 2 tablespoons cocoa powder

60g non-dairy chocolate chips or chopped chocolate

¾ teaspoon fine-grain sea salt

1½ teaspoons baking powder

175ml almond milk

2 tablespoons coconut oil, melted

1½ teaspoons pure vanilla extract

300ml hot coffee (decaf, if desired) or boiled water

Vegan ice cream, for serving (optional)

Icing sugar, for serving (optional)

Toasted walnuts, for serving (optional)

Pudding cake magically creates its own thick chocolate sauce on the bottom of the dish while it bakes. It's like eating a warm chocolate pudding with pieces of chocolate cake mixed throughout. My sister Kristi calls this cake a 'melt in your mouth chocolate explosion!' If you've never made a pudding cake before, you might be nervous when the cake comes out of the oven because it won't look like it has baked for enough time. The truth is, a pudding cake *should* look underdone when it comes out of the oven – the sides of the cake will be bubbly with chocolate sauce and the top of the cake will be firm in some places and gooey in others. This is totally normal and not a cause for alarm. This recipe calls for brewed coffee (regular or decaf), but if you are serving it to kids or you don't like a subtle coffee flavour, you can use boiled water instead. I like to use freshly brewed French press coffee, but 1 teaspoon instant coffee mixed with boiling water also works in a pinch. This cake is lovely with a scoop of vegan ice cream and a sprinkle of toasted walnuts for some added crunch.

Makes 9 servings

PREP TIME: 15 minutes • BAKE TIME: 28 to 34 minutes
gluten-free, refined sugar-free, nut-free option, soy-free option

1. Preheat the oven to 190°C (375°F). Lightly grease a 2-litre square glass baking dish.

2. In a small bowl, whisk the flaxseed and 3 tablespoons water together. Set aside.

3. In a large bowl, mix together the oat flour, 170g of the sugar, 60g of the cocoa powder, and the chocolate chips, salt, and baking powder.

4. In a small bowl, whisk together the flaxseed mixture, almond milk, oil, and vanilla.

5. Pour the milk mixture over the flour mixture and stir until thoroughly combined.

6. Pour the batter into the prepared baking dish and smooth out the top evenly with a spoon.

7. In a small bowl or mug, combine the remaining sugar and remaining 2 tablespoons of cocoa powder. Sprinkle the mixture evenly over the batter in the baking dish.

8. Slowly pour the hot coffee over the cocoa powder mixture, ensuring that the coffee completely covers the mixture. The cake will now look like a complete disaster, but this is normal. Promise.

9. Bake for 27 to 33 minutes, uncovered, until the cake is semi-firm on top but bubbly and gooey around the edges.

10. Let the cake cool for 5 to 10 minutes before digging in (that's if you can wait that long!). If desired, serve with vegan ice cream, along with a dusting of icing sugar and toasted walnuts on top.

Tips: For a nut-free option, swap out the almond milk for a nut-free non-dairy milk (such as coconut milk) and leave out the optional walnuts.

For a soy-free option, use soy-free non-dairy chocolate, such as Enjoy Life brand.

gluten-free chocolate-almond brownies

4 teaspoons ground flaxseed

140g whole raw almonds

115g plus 2 tablespoons brown rice flour

2 tablespoons arrowroot powder

50g cocoa powder, sifted

½ teaspoon kosher salt

¼ teaspoon baking soda

90g plus 45g non-dairy chocolate chips

55g plus 2 tablespoons vegan butter or coconut oil

225g natural cane sugar

60ml almond milk

1 teaspoon pure vanilla extract

65g finely chopped walnuts (optional)

I went through many trials to test these gluten-free and vegan brownies. It was no easy feat! Many of my trials turned out too fluffy and cake-like – two characteristics that I'm not looking for in a brownie. Finally, I struck it rich with this amazing recipe. These brownies are dense and chewy, just the way a brownie should be, and I can promise, you'll never know they are gluten-free and vegan.

Makes 16 small squares

PREP TIME: 30 minutes   •   COOK TIME: 30 to 36 minutes
gluten-free, soy-free option, refined sugar-free

1. Preheat the oven to 180°C (350°F). Lightly oil a 2.5-litre square cake pan and line it with two pieces of parchment paper, one going each way.

2. In a small bowl, whisk together the flaxseed and 3 tablespoons of water and set aside.

3. In a blender or food processor, grind the almonds into a meal/ flour. Sift out any large pieces. In a large bowl, whisk together the ground almonds, brown rice flour, arrowroot, cocoa powder, salt, and baking soda.

4. In a medium saucepan, melt 90g of the chocolate chips and the vegan butter over low heat. When two-thirds of the chips have melted, remove the pan from the heat and stir until smooth. Stir in the flaxseed mixture, sugar, almond milk, and vanilla until combined.

5. Pour the chocolate mixture over the ground almond mixture and stir well until there's no flour on the bottom of the bowl. Fold in the walnuts, if desired, and the remaining chocolate chips.

6. Spoon the batter into the prepared pan and place a piece of

parchment on top. Press down on the parchment paper with your hands to spread out the batter. Use a pastry roller to even it out, if desired.

7. Bake for 28 to 34 minutes. Let the brownies cool in the pan for 1 to 1½ hours. Do not remove the brownies until they are completely cool or they will crumble. After cooling, slice the brownies into squares and enjoy with a glass of Creamy Vanilla Almond Milk (see page 277). The brownies will stay fresh in an airtight container for up to 3 days.

Tips: If you don't want to make gluten-free brownies, feel free to omit the brown rice flour and arrowroot powder and replace them with 90g unbleached all-purpose flour. Use the 140g almonds as stated in the recipe.

For a soy-free option, use soy-free chocolate, such as Enjoy Life brand.

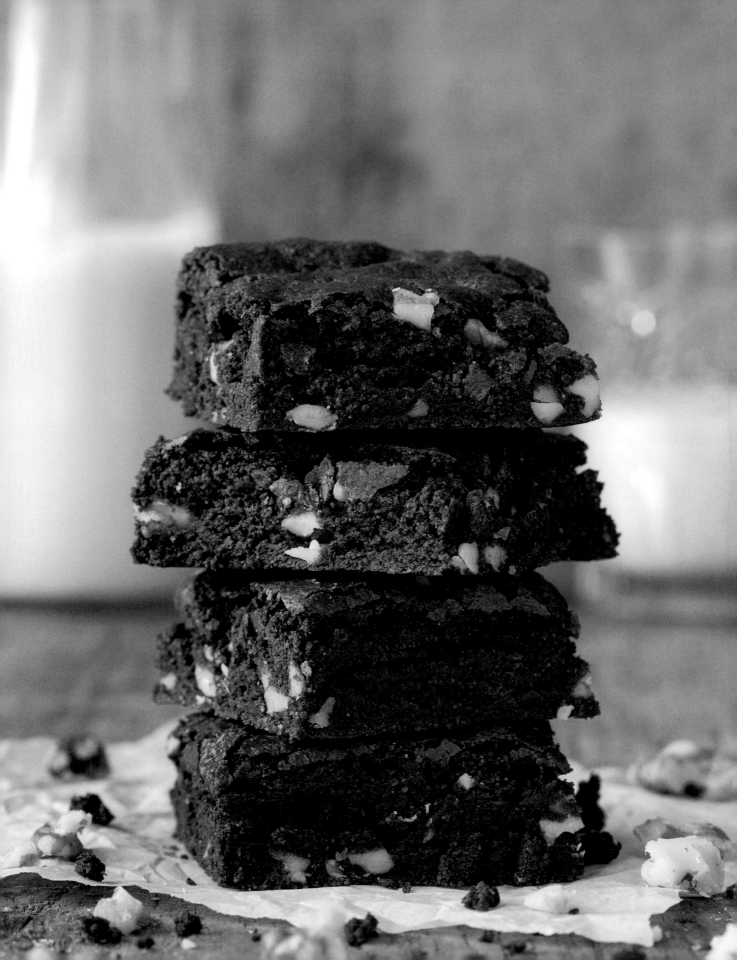

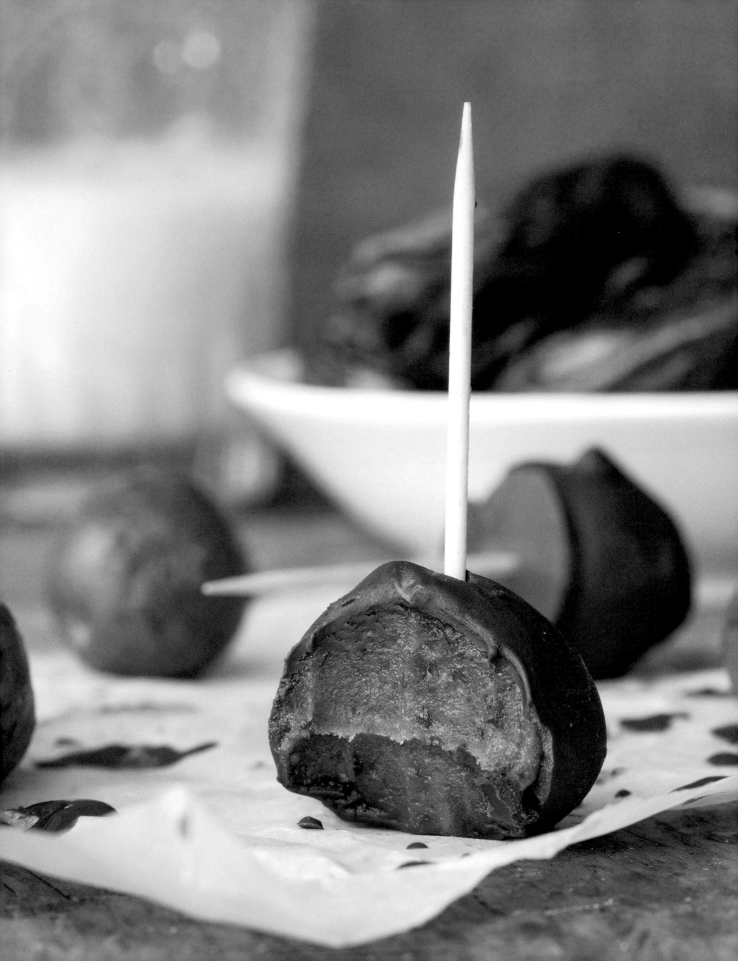

homemade yolos

FOR THE CARAMEL:
200g pitted soft Medjool dates

1½ teaspoons peanut butter or other nut or seed butter

Pinch of fine-grain sea salt

FOR THE CHOCOLATE COATING:
45g plus 3 tablespoons dark chocolate chips

½ teaspoon coconut oil

Flaked sea salt or chia seeds (optional)

This candy recipe is inspired by one of my favorite store-bought candies growing up. I bet you can take a wild guess what they were! The buttery caramel made by Medjool dates will remind you so much of the real candy that your head will spin. People often tell me these homemade Yolos are better than the real thing! I would have to agree. Hey, you only live once!

Makes 20 Yolos

PREP TIME: 25 minutes • CHILL TIME: 40 minutes

gluten-free, raw/no-bake, soy-free option, grain-free, nut-free option

1. Make the Caramel: Process the pitted dates in a food processor until a sticky paste forms. Add the peanut butter and salt and process until combined. The mixture will be very sticky, but this is what we want.

2. Scoop the sticky mixture into a bowl and freeze, uncovered, for about 10 minutes. (Chilling makes the caramel easier to shape into balls.) Line a plate with parchment paper. Lightly wet your fingers and shape the chilled caramel into small balls, making about 20 in total. Set the balls on the parchment paper-lined plate as you roll them. Place the finished balls in the freezer for 10 minutes to firm up.

3. Make the Chocolate Coating: In a small saucepan, melt the chocolate chips and oil over very low heat. When two-thirds of the chips have melted, remove the pan from the heat and stir until smooth.

4. Remove the caramel balls from the freezer and dunk each ball into the melted chocolate, one at a time. Roll them around with a fork to coat. Tap off any excess chocolate coating and set the balls back on the lined plate. If desired, stick a toothpick in the top of

each ball and sprinkle the balls with a tiny amount of flaked sea salt or chia seeds.

5. Freeze the balls for at least 20 minutes, or until the chocolate is set. Yolos taste best straight from the freezer and will soften at room temperature.

Tips: If your dates are stiff or dry, soak them in water for 30 to 60 minutes to soften them before use. Drain them well and blot off excess water before processing. If you have leftover melted chocolate, scoop it onto a parchment paper-lined plate and freeze it. The chocolate will harden back up and you won't have to throw any away. Break up the chocolate and store it for another use. Waste not, want not, as my mother always says!

For a nut-free option, use sunflower seed butter instead of nut butter.

For a soy-free option, use soy-free non-diary chocolate (such as Enjoy Life brand).

crispy almond butter chocolate chip cookies

1 tablespoon ground flaxseed

25g vegan butter or 60ml coconut oil

65g roasted almond butter or peanut butter

100g Sucanat sugar or brown sugar

55g coconut sugar or natural cane sugar

1 teaspoon pure vanilla extract

½ teaspoon baking soda

½ teaspoon baking powder

½ teaspoon fine-grain sea salt

100g gluten-free rolled oats, blended into a flour

120g almonds, blended into almond meal

45g mini dark chocolate chips or finely chopped dark chocolate

These crispy around the edges, chewy, and nutty chocolate chip cookies are made with almonds and oats so they are naturally gluten-free. Try them yourself and see why they are a fan-favourite on my blog.

Makes 16 to 20 cookies

PREP TIME: 20 minutes • BAKE TIME: 12 to 14 minutes

gluten-free, refined sugar-free, soy-free option,
grain-free option, nut-free option

1. Preheat the oven to 180°C (350°F). Line a baking sheet with parchment paper.

2. In a small bowl, mix together the flaxseed and 3 tablespoons of water and set aside for 5 minutes to thicken.

3. With a hand mixer or in the bowl of a stand mixer fitted with the paddle attachment, beat together the vegan butter and almond butter until combined. Add both sugars and beat for 1 minute more. Beat in the flaxseed mixture and vanilla until combined.

4. One by one, beat in the baking soda, baking powder, salt, oat flour, and almond meal. The dough should be lightly sticky. If your dough is dry, you can add a touch of almond milk to thin it out. Fold in the chocolate chips.

5. Shape the dough into 2.5cm balls. If the chocolate chips aren't sticking to the dough, just press them in with your fingers. Place the balls on the prepared baking sheet as you roll them, leaving 5 to 8cm of space between them. There is no need to flatten the balls as the cookies spread out as they bake.

6. Bake for 12 to 14 minutes, until golden brown on the bottom. The cookies will be very soft coming out of the oven, but they will harden

as they cool. Let cool for 5 minutes on the baking sheet and then transfer to a cooling rack to cool for 10 minutes more. I like to store these in the freezer so they stay nice and crispy.

Tips: If an entire batch of these is too tempting to have around the house, simply freeze balls of uncooked dough for a later use. Whenever the cookie craving strikes, just thaw the dough for 30 to 60 minutes on the counter and bake as usual.

For a grain-free option, omit the rolled oats and use 235g whole almonds (ground into a meal). Bake at 160°C (325°F) for 13 to 15 minutes.

For a soy-free option, use soy-free vegan butter or coconut oil and soy-free chocolate chips (such as Enjoy Life brand).

For a nut-free option, swap out the nut butter for sunflower seed butter and swap out the almonds for an extra 50g plus 1 tablespoon rolled oats. In other words, you will use 100g plus 50g plus 1 tablespoon rolled oats total. Grind the oats into a flour.

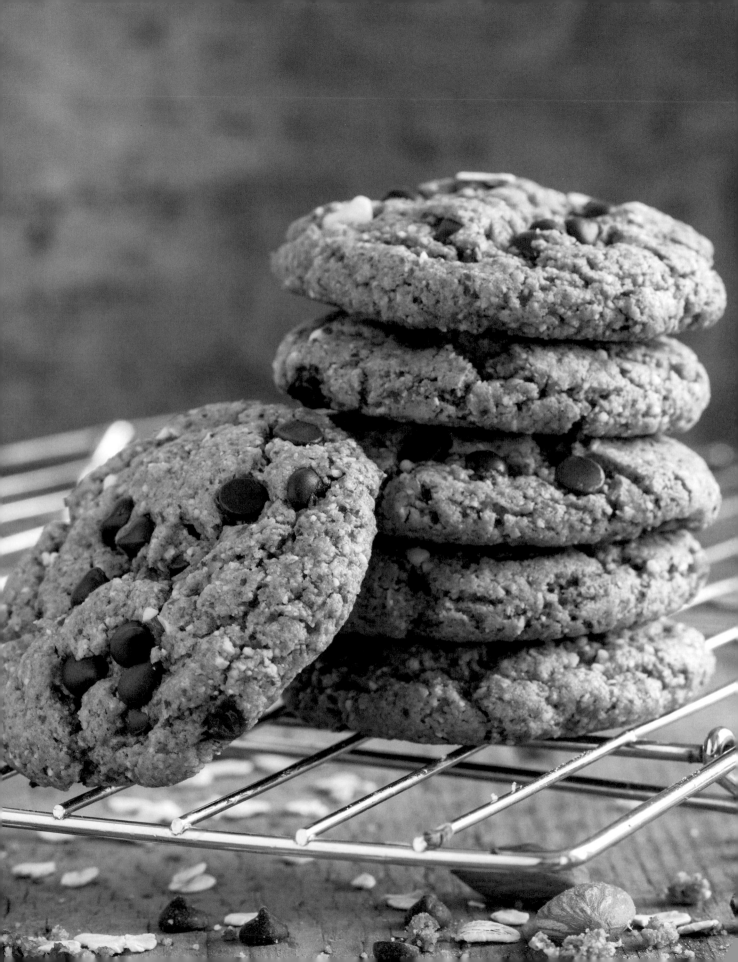

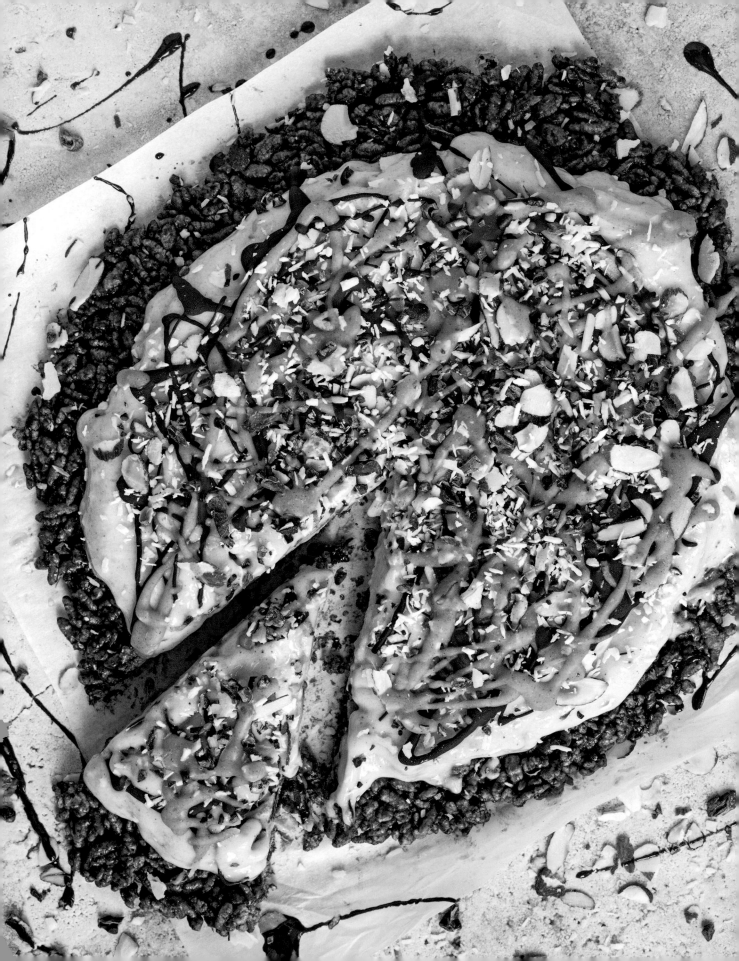

beat the heat frozen dessert pizza

FOR THE CRUST:

50g rice crisp cereal

2 tablespoons plus 1½ teaspoons brown rice syrup or coconut nectar syrup

2 tablespoons coconut oil, melted

4 teaspoons cocoa powder

1 batch Banana Soft Serve (see page 289)

TOPPINGS:

60g dark chocolate chips

2 teaspoons coconut oil

1 tablespoon roasted almond butter or peanut butter

1 tablespoon coconut oil, softened

1 teaspoon pure maple syrup

4 teaspoons toasted sliced almonds

2 teaspoons cacao nibs or chopped chocolate

1 tablespoon shredded unsweetened coconut

Growing up, my sister and I always requested a certain popular frozen dessert pizza on our birthdays. This is my vegan, healthier take on it. I don't miss the store-bought version one bit! Be sure to freeze the bananas the night before so that they are ready when you make the pizza.

Makes 10 to 12 servings

PREP TIME: 25 to 30 minutes • FREEZE TIME: 15 to 20 minutes

gluten-free, soy-free option, raw/no-bake

1. Line a pizza pan with a circle of parchment paper.

2. Make the Crust: In a large bowl, mix the cereal, brown rice syrup, oil, and cocoa powder until all the cereal is coated. Spoon the crust mixture onto the prepared pizza pan and spread it out into a 25cm circle. Add a piece of parchment paper on top and press down with your hands to compact the mixture and form the shape. Place the pan in the freezer for 5 to 10 minutes, until firm.

3. Gently spread the Banana Soft Serve over the chilled crust, leaving about 2.5cm around the edge. Return the pan to the freezer for 5 to 10 minutes.

4. For the Toppings: In a small saucepan, melt the chocolate chips and 2 teaspoons of the oil over very low heat. When two-thirds of the chips have melted, remove the pan from the heat and stir until completely smooth.

5. In a small bowl, stir together the almond butter, remaining 1 tablespoon oil, and the maple syrup. Transfer the mixture to a small plastic bag and snip off the corner so you can 'pipe' it onto the pizza.

6. Drizzle one-third of the melted chocolate over the pizza and 'pipe' on one-third of the almond butter mixture. Immediately sprinkle the pizza with half of the sliced almonds, cocoa nibs, and coconut. Repeat this entire step until you don't have any toppings left.

7. Return the pizza to the freezer for 5 to 10 minutes more, then slice and serve immediately. This pizza is best enjoyed frozen, straight from the freezer, and will melt quickly.

Tips: Instead of the Banana Soft Serve, you can substitute 220g of your favorite non-dairy ice cream.

Feel free to get creative and use any toppings you desire. The sky is the limit!

For a soy-free option, use soy-free non-dairy chocolate (such as Enjoy Life brand).

homemade staples

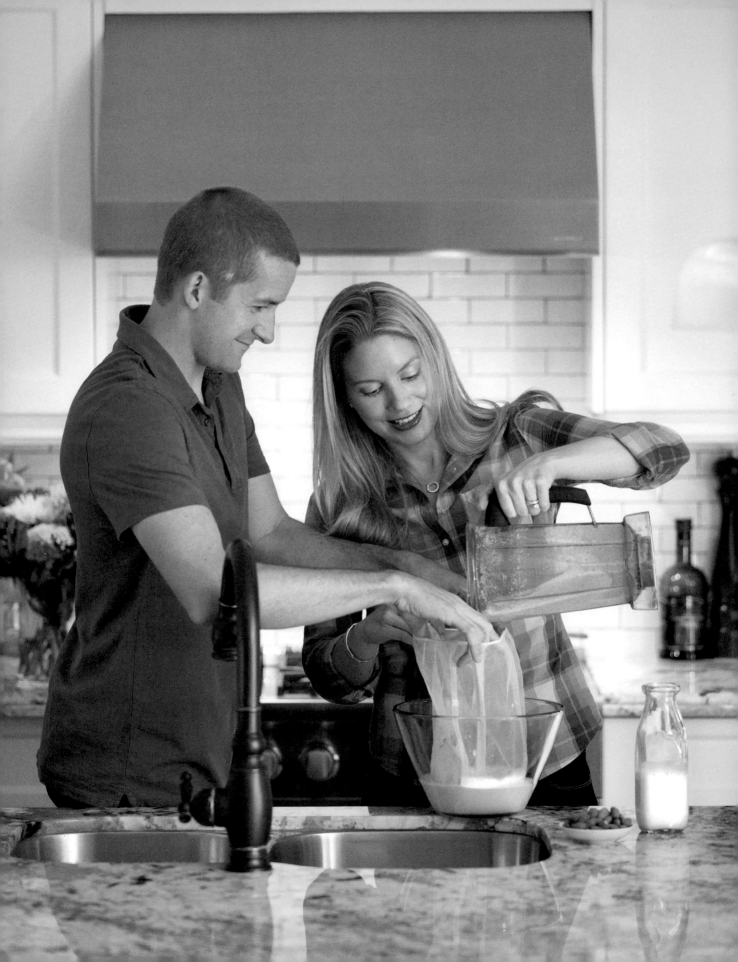

This chapter includes quick and easy staple recipes that I try to make at home as much as possible. I'm a firm believer that everything tastes better when it's homemade, and it's easier on the wallet. That isn't to say that I don't rely on store-bought goods from time to time, because I certainly do, but I love rolling up my sleeves and making these staples myself whenever I can. In this chapter you'll find recipes for almond milk, gluten-free croutons, vegetable broth, nut butter, mayonnaise, breadcrumbs, enchilada sauce, gravy, salad dressing, and so much more. You'll also find simple instructions for making whole grain and nut flours in your blender, as well as methods for roasting garlic and pressing tofu. In today's busy world, getting back to the basics can feel like a daunting task, but there's a certain sense of satisfaction that comes from making things from scratch. I hope you'll be inspired to try out a few of these yourself!

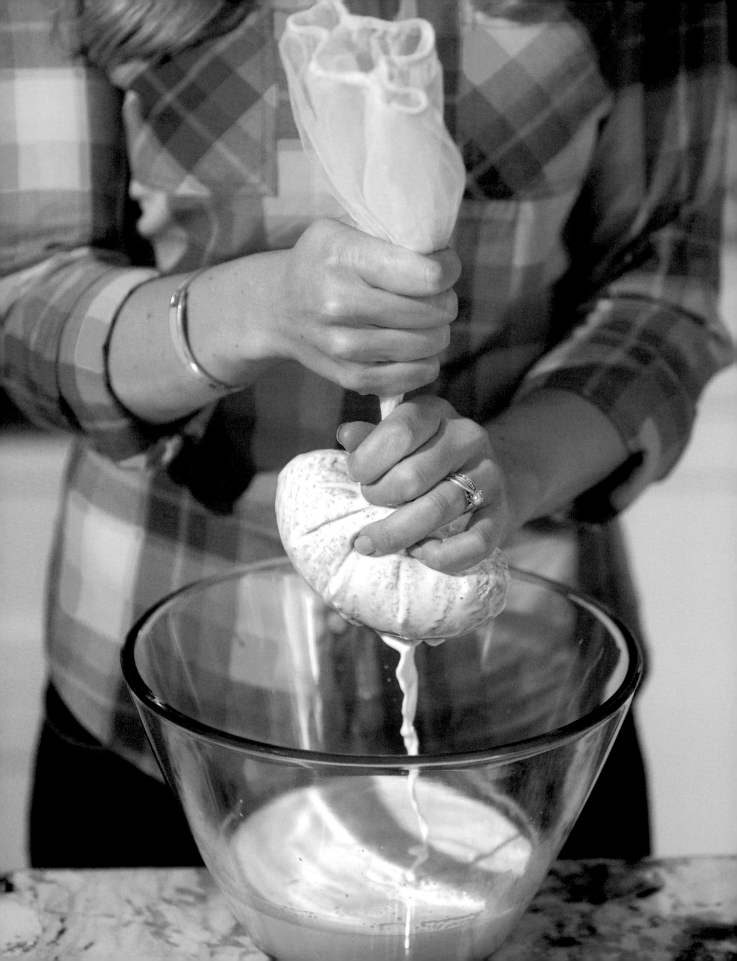

creamy vanilla almond milk

140g raw almonds

1 litre filtered water (or try coconut water for a fun twist)

2 to 3 soft Medjool dates, pitted, or liquid sweetener to taste

1 vanilla bean, roughly chopped, or ½ to 1 teaspoon pure vanilla extract, to taste

¼ teaspoon ground cinnamon

Pinch of fine-grain sea salt

Tips: If your dates or vanilla bean are dry/stiff, soak them in water to soften before use.

Reserve the pulp left in the bag for making Easy Almond Pulp Granola (page 276).

For a long time, I thought making almond milk at home would be a drawn-out, complicated process. Then I discovered just how easy and delicious it really is. Once you soak raw almonds overnight, all you need to do is blend them with water and strain them through a nut milk bag. It's so easy, and the flavour beats store-bought almond milk by a landslide! A nut milk bag is my preferred method of straining out the pulp, but you may also have success using a fine-mesh strainer and cheesecloth.

Makes 1 litre

PREP TIME: 10 minutes

gluten-free, oil-free, raw/no-bake, soy-free, sugar-free, grain-free

1. Place the almonds in a bowl and add enough water to cover by an inch or two. Soak the almonds overnight (for 8 to 12 hours), preferably, but you can get away with soaking for 1 to 2 hours in a pinch.

2. Drain and rinse the almonds very well. Place them in a blender along with the water, dates, vanilla bean, cinnamon, and salt and blend on high for about 1 minute.

3. Place a nut milk bag over a large bowl and slowly pour the almond mixture into the bag. Gently squeeze the bottom of the bag to release the milk. It can take 3 to 5 minutes to release all of the milk, so be patient.

4. Carefully pour the milk into a glass jar. Homemade almond milk will keep in the refrigerator for 3 to 4 days. The milk separates while sitting, so be sure to give the jar a good shake before using.

easy almond pulp granola

60g to 120g almond pulp, left over from making Creamy Vanilla Almond Milk (see page 275)

100g gluten-free rolled oats

½ to 1 teaspoon ground cinnamon, to taste

1 teaspoon pure vanilla extract

3 to 4 tablespoons pure maple syrup or sweetener of choice, to taste

Pinch of fine-grain sea salt

This recipe is a quick and easy way to use up the almond pulp left over from making Creamy Vanilla Almond Milk (page 275). Just mix everything together in one bowl and place it in a dehydrator overnight. The next morning, you'll wake up to delicious, crunchy granola to enjoy with your homemade almond milk. And a word of caution: You really do need to use a dehydrator for this recipe; I did not have much success using a traditional oven.

Makes 600ml

PREP TIME: 5 minutes

oil-free, refined sugar-free, soy-free, gluten-free

1. Line a dehydrator tray with a non-stick dehydrator sheet.

2. In a medium bowl, combine all of the ingredients. Spread the mixture on the dehydrator sheet in a thin layer.

3. Dehydrate the granola for 11 to 12 hours at 45°C (115°F), or until dry and crispy. Serve with homemade almond milk (see page 275), in a parfait, or sprinkled over Effortless Vegan Overnight Oats (see page 29).

almond meal

In a blender or food processor, blend/process 140g whole raw almonds on high until they have a flour-like consistency. The texture should be like that of coarse flour, but not as fine as regular flour. Be sure not to blend the almonds for too long or the oils will start to release and the meal will stick together in clumps. If this happens, simply break apart the clumps with your fingers. Before using, sift out any large pieces of almonds.

almond flour

In a blender or food processor, blend/process 140g blanched whole almonds on high speed until a flour forms. Be sure not to blend for too long or the oils will release and the flour may clump together. Sift out any clumps or large almond pieces before using.

oat flour

In a blender, blend your desired amount of rolled oats on high speed for several seconds, until they have a fine, flour-like consistency.

raw buckwheat flour

In a blender, blend your desired amount of raw buckwheat groats on high speed until they have a fine, flour-like consistency.

grapeseed mayonnaise

250ml grapeseed oil

125ml plain unsweetened soy milk (no substitutes)

1 teaspoon apple cider vinegar

1 tablespoon fresh lemon juice

1 teaspoon brown rice syrup

¼ teaspoon dry mustard

¾ teaspoon fine-grain sea salt

When I see a fairly short ingredients list on one of my favourite store-bought foods, I usually try to see if I can make it at home. As it turns out, vegan mayonnaise is incredibly easy and quick to make at home. I simply looked at the ingredients label of my favorite vegan mayonnaise and started to experiment with ingredient quantities. After a few trials, I think this version hits the nail on the head. I hope you enjoy it, too!

Makes 325ml

PREP TIME: 5 minutes

gluten-free, nut-free, refined sugar-free, raw/no-bake, grain-free

1. In a high-speed blender, combine all of the ingredients except the oil and blend on high until smooth, stopping to scrape down the sides of the blender cup as necessary. Slowly stream in the oil through the blender top while blending. The mixture will thicken gradually.

2. Transfer to an airtight container and refrigerate. The mayonnaise will keep for up to 1 month.

Tip: I do not recommend subbing any other kind of non-dairy milk for the soy milk, as its protein content helps with thickening. I didn't have any luck using almond milk (it was a runny mess).

sprouted-grain breadcrumbs

3 slices sprouted-grain bread (or bread of choice)

These sprouted-grain breadcrumbs are not only healthy and easy to make, but they last for a month or longer in an airtight container. I like to keep a batch of these on hand to save myself from buying store-bought breadcrumbs. It's also a great solution if you find yourself with a stale loaf of bread – instead of throwing out the bread, why not transform it into breadcrumbs? Be sure to make these in advance, as they need to sit out overnight to dry.

Makes 120g

PREP TIME: 5 minutes • COOK TIME: 5 to 10 minutes

nut-free, oil-free, soy-free, sugar-free

1. Place the bread in a toaster and toast until lightly browned (but not burned). (I toast the bread a bit darker than I normally would without completely charring it.)

2. Transfer to a cooling rack and cool for 15 minutes.

3. Tear the bread into chunks and place them in a food processor. Process until a fine crumb the texture of coarse sand forms.

4. Line a baking sheet with parchment paper. Spread out the crumbs in a single layer on the sheet and leave to dry out, uncovered, overnight (or for at least 8 hours).

5. Store the breadcrumbs in an airtight container for 4 to 8 weeks.

whipped coconut cream

1 396g can full-fat coconut milk

1 to 2 tablespoons sweetener, to taste

1 vanilla bean, seeds scraped, or
½ teaspoon pure vanilla extract

Did you know you can make a decadent, fluffy whipped cream by using a can of full-fat coconut milk? Not only is it simple to make, but it's easily the best-tasting whipped cream I've tried. You can use this whipped cream just like regular dairy whipped cream. I like to use it as a garnish for desserts (like my Raw Pumpkin-Maple Pie on page 247), and it's also amazing with a bowl of fruit, on top of a fruit crisp, or stirred into Banana Soft Serve (see page 289). The options are really endless!

Makes 175ml to 250ml
PREP TIME: 5 to 10 minutes
gluten-free, nut-free, oil-free, refined sugar-free,
soy-free, grain-free, raw/no-bake

1. Chill the can of coconut milk in the fridge overnight (or for at least 9 to 10 hours).

2. About 1 hour before making the whipped cream, chill a bowl in the freezer.

3. Flip the chilled can upside down and open it with a can opener. Pour off the coconut water (you can reserve it for smoothies if you'd like).

4. Scoop the solid coconut cream into the chilled bowl.

5. Using an electric hand mixer, beat the cream until fluffy and smooth. Add the sweetener (maple syrup, agave nectar, or even natural cane sugar) and the vanilla bean seeds and beat gently just to combine.

6. Cover the bowl and return the whipped cream to the fridge until ready to use. It will firm when chilled and soften at room temperature. The whipped cream will keep in a sealed container in the refrigerator for 1 to 2 weeks.

oh she glows

For Coconut-Lemon Whipped Cream: Whip the coconut cream and add 1 tablespoon fresh lemon juice and 2 tablespoons sweetener of choice.

For Chocolate Fudge Whipped Cream: Whip the coconut cream and add 3 to 4 tablespoons sifted cocoa powder, 2 tablespoons sweetener of choice, ¼ teaspoon pure vanilla extract, and a pinch of fine-grain sea salt.

cashew cream

Cashew cream can be used in a variety of recipes as a substitute for dairy cream or even sour cream.

In a bowl, combine 150g raw cashews and enough water to cover them and soak for 8 hours or overnight (for a quick-soak method, put the cashews in a bowl, pour boiling water over them until the cashews are covered, and soak for 2 hours). Drain and rinse the cashews and transfer them to a blender with 125ml to 250ml water. Less water will give you a thicker sauce. Blend on high speed until the cream is smooth. If using the cashew cream for a savoury recipe, add a pinch of salt, if desired.

To make Cashew Sour Cream, add the following ingredients to the blender with the cashews and water and blend on high speed until smooth:

    2 teaspoons fresh lemon juice

    1 teaspoon apple cider vinegar

    ½ teaspoon plus ⅛ teaspoon fine-grain sea salt, or to taste

easy mushroom gravy

1½ teaspoons extra-virgin olive oil

1 sweet or yellow onion, finely chopped

2 large cloves garlic, minced

Fine-grain sea salt and freshly ground black pepper

230g sliced cremini mushrooms

1 teaspoon minced fresh rosemary

2 tablespoons plus 1½ teaspoons all-purpose flour

300ml vegetable broth

2 tablespoons low-sodium tamari, or to taste

This is a simple, yet satisfying, gravy that comes together in no time. It's great for holiday meals, and we love to pour it on top of Cauliflower Mashed Potatoes (see page 207).

Makes 500ml

PREP TIME: 5 minutes • COOK TIME: 10 minutes

gluten-free option, nut-free, sugar-free, soy-free option

1. In a frying pan or saucepan, heat the oil over a medium heat. Add the onion and garlic and sauté for 3 to 4 minutes. Season with salt and pepper.

2. Add the sliced mushrooms and rosemary and raise the heat to medium-high. Sauté for 8 to 9 minutes more, or until most of the water released by the mushrooms has cooked off.

3. Stir in the flour until all the vegetables are coated.

4. Add the broth and tamari gradually and stir quickly to smooth out any clumps of flour. Bring the mixture to a simmer. Cook, stirring often to ensure that it doesn't burn, for 5 minutes more.

5. When the gravy has thickened to your liking, remove the pan from the heat and serve.

Tip: For a gluten-free option, use all-purpose gluten-free flour and gluten-free tamari. For a soy-free option, use coconut aminos in place of tamari.

If at any point the gravy becomes too thick, simply thin it out with a bit more broth. Likewise, if it's too thin, thicken it with a bit more flour.

effortless anytime
balsamic vinaigrette

60ml apple cider vinegar

3 tablespoons flaxseed oil or extra-virgin olive oil

2 tablespoons balsamic vinegar

2 tablespoons unsweetened applesauce

1 tablespoon pure maple syrup

1½ teaspoons Dijon mustard

1 clove garlic, minced

¼ teaspoon fine-grain sea salt, or to taste

Freshly ground black pepper

Salad dressing doesn't get much quicker than this! This dressing stores well in the fridge and is a great alternative to store-bought salad dressing. I just toss everything into a mason jar, screw on the lid, and shake it up! My favourite way to enjoy it is mixed with courgette pasta; I've been known to spiralize an entire courgette, cover it with this dressing, and devour it in minutes. It's also fantastic in my Walnut, Avocado & Pear Salad (see page 103).

Makes 175ml

PREP TIME: 5 minutes

*gluten-free, nut-free, raw/no-bake,
soy-free, refined sugar-free, grain-free*

1. In a small bowl, whisk together all of the ingredients or simply combine them in a jar, screw on the lid, and shake. This dressing will keep in an airtight container in the fridge for at least 2 weeks.

Tip: Feel free to adjust this dressing to suit your own taste preferences. I tend to like an acidic bite to my salad dressing, but if you prefer less acidity, simply decrease the vinegar or increase the sweetener. Have fun and play around with the amounts!

lemon-tahini dressing

1 large clove garlic

60ml tahini

60ml fresh lemon juice

3 tablespoons nutritional yeast

1 to 2 tablespoons sesame oil or extra-virgin olive oil, to taste

1 to 2 tablespoons water

¼ teaspoon fine-grain sea salt, or to taste

Quite possibly one of my all-time favourite salad dressings, this creamy, tangy dressing works well in a variety of dishes like my Oil-Free Baked Falafel Bites (see page 95).

Makes 150ml

PREP TIME: 5 minutes

gluten-free, nut-free, raw/no-bake, soy-free, sugar-free, grain-free

1. In a food processor, pulse the garlic to mince it. Add the tahini, lemon juice, nutritional yeast, oil, water, and salt and process until smooth.

Tip: The dressing will thicken up a bit once chilled. Feel free to thin it out, if necessary, with a tablespoon or two of water or oil.

10-spice blend

2 tablespoons smoked paprika

1 tablespoon garlic powder

1 tablespoon dried oregano

1 tablespoon onion powder

1 tablespoon dried basil

2 teaspoons dried thyme

1½ teaspoons freshly ground black pepper

1½ teaspoons fine-grain sea salt

1 teaspoon white pepper

1 teaspoon cayenne pepper

This spice blend takes less than five minutes to throw together, and it can be used in a variety of dishes, from soups and stews to baked potatoes, kale chips, tofu, beans, avocado toast and more. Try it in my 10-Spice Vegetable Soup with Cashew Cream for a flavourful soup that's sure to dazzle your taste buds (see page 137).

Makes 125ml

PREP TIME: 5 minutes

gluten-free, raw/no-bake, sugar-free, oil-free, soy-free, grain-free

1. Combine all of the ingredients in a medium jar. Secure the lid and shake to combine. Shake the jar before each use.

pressed tofu

When I first started to experiment with tofu, I had no idea what all of this 'pressing' talk was about. *Why do I need to press tofu? It looks pretty firm already!* Well, I soon found out that there's a lot of water hiding inside tofu blocks (yes, even in the firm and extra-firm varieties). Pressing the tofu helps release unnecessary water, resulting in a firmer, denser block of tofu.

Stack-and-tumble method

If you don't have a tofu press, here's the old-fashioned (and free!) method of pressing tofu. Just be warned, the books like to tumble over at the slightest breeze.

Rinse the tofu. Cover a cutting board with a couple of kitchen towels. Wrap the tofu with a few sheets of paper towel and then wrap it with a thick kitchen towel. Place the tofu on top of the cutting board and add another towel on top of the tofu. Set several heavy cookbooks on top. Let the books sit on the tofu for at least 20 minutes to press out the water. Just be sure to keep an eye on it; those cookbooks like to tumble over! It's best if you can secure the stack between a wall and a large appliance.

Tofu press

After a couple of years of using the stacking method, I finally started to use a tofu press. It changed everything! The tofu press gets out much more water (with no tumbling books!). I love to let the tofu press do its thing overnight in the fridge for a super-duper-firm tofu. It collects the water at the bottom and I'm always shocked by how much it presses out of the tofu. If you are a regular tofu consumer, it's a great investment and won't take up much space at all. My brand of choice is Tofu Xpress.

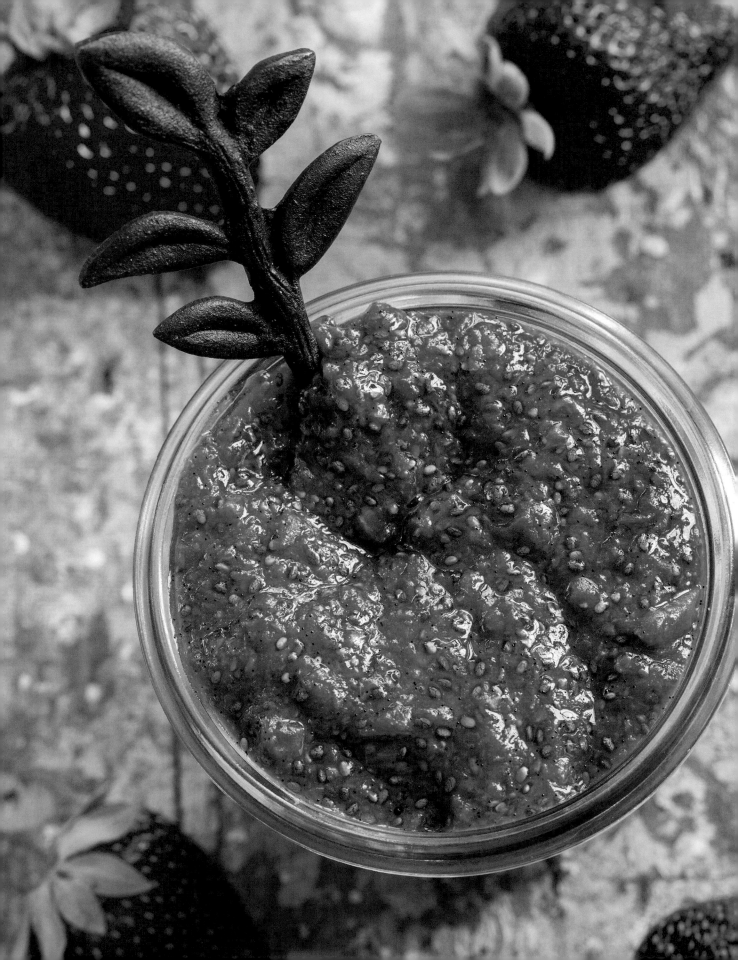

magical chia seed jam

600g fresh or frozen raspberries, blackberries, blueberries, or strawberries

3 to 4 tablespoons pure maple syrup or other sweetener, to taste

2 tablespoons chia seeds

1 teaspoon pure vanilla extract

Tip: If making strawberry chia seed jam, process the hulled strawberries in a food processor until almost smooth. The strawberries don't break down as quickly as other berries do, so this helps them along. After processing, simply transfer the strawberry mixture to a saucepan and proceed with cooking as usual.

If you've got twenty minutes, you can make a healthy jam that will rival any store-bought jam. All you do is cook down fruit (blueberries, raspberries, strawberries, etc.) with chia seeds and a touch of sweetener until it thickens up. You won't believe how thick this gets – hence, the name Magical Chia Seed Jam! Thanks to the chia seeds, we're also pumping up the jam with all kinds of healthy omega-3 fatty acids, iron, fibre, protein, magnesium, and calcium. Who knew jam could be so healthy?

Makes 250ml

PREP TIME: 20 minutes • CHILL TIME: 2 hours
gluten-free, oil-free, refined sugar-free, soy-free, nut-free, grain-free

1. In a medium saucepan, combine the berries and 3 tablespoons of the maple syrup and bring to a simmer over a medium to high heat, stirring frequently. Reduce the heat to medium-low and simmer for about 5 minutes. Lightly mash the berries with a potato masher or fork, leaving some whole for texture.

2. Stir in the chia seeds until thoroughly combined and cook, stirring frequently, until the mixture thickens to your desired consistency, or about 15 minutes.

3. Once the jam is thick, remove the pan from the heat and stir in the vanilla. Add more sweetener to taste, if desired. Enjoy on toast, English muffins, oatmeal, Effortless Vegan Overnight Oats (see page 37), oat bars, tarts, cookies, Banana Soft Serve (see page 289), and more. The jam should keep in an airtight container in the fridge for 1 to 2 weeks and it will thicken up even more as it cools.

chocolate frosting (two ways)

CHOCOLATE BUTTERCREAM:
Makes 500ml

315g icing sugar, sifted

75g cocoa powder, sifted

115g vegan butter (such as Earth Balance)

Pinch of fine-grain sea salt

2 teaspoons pure vanilla extract

3½ to 4 tablespoons non-dairy milk, as needed

CHOCOLATE-AVOCADO FROSTING:
Makes 375ml

2 large ripe avocados, pitted

6 tablespoons unsweetened cocoa powder, sifted

5 to 6 tablespoons agave nectar, to taste

2 teaspoons pure vanilla extract

Pinch of fine-grain sea salt

Here are two delicious, rich chocolate frosting recipes to choose from. The Chocolate Buttercream is classic in flavour and a great all-purpose frosting, while the Chocolate-Avocado Frosting is less sweet with an intense, creamy dark chocolate base.

FOR THE CHOCOLATE BUTTERCREAM:

1. With a hand mixer, beat all the ingredients except the milk together in a large bowl. Add the milk gradually. You want the texture to be thick, but not so thick that it won't spread, and not runny. You may need to use more or less milk than stated, but 3½ tablespoons was perfect for me.

FOR THE CHOCOLATE-AVOCADO FROSTING:

1. In a food processor, process the avocado until mostly smooth. Add the rest of the ingredients and process again until smooth, scraping down the bowl as needed.

2. Transfer to the fridge until ready to use. The frosting will keep in an airtight container in the fridge for up to 3 days.

banana soft serve

4 ripe bananas, peeled, chopped, and frozen

2 tablespoons roasted almond butter or peanut butter (optional)

I first heard about Banana Soft Serve from my talented friend Gena Hamshaw, who writes the blog choosingraw.com. It forever changed the way I looked at soft-serve ice cream! It's a healthy treat that I make on a regular basis, and it's a great pick-me-up on a hot summer day. The sky is the limit when it comes to what you can add into this treat. Frozen berries, nut butter, cacao nibs, cocoa or carob powder are all very tasty additions. In the summer, I try to always have some frozen bananas on hand, just for this very recipe.

Serves 2

PREP TIME: 5 minutes

gluten-free, nut-free option, soy-free,
sugar-free, grain-free, raw/no-bake, oil-free

1. In a food processor, process the frozen bananas and almond butter (if using) until smooth, stopping to scrape down the sides of the bowl as necessary. This process can take several minutes, depending on your food processor.

2. When the banana mixture is smooth and has the consistency of soft-serve ice cream, remove it from the processor and enjoy immediately.

Tip: I recommend using yellow bananas with only a few spots. If the bananas are too ripe and spotted, they do not get as creamy and also have a very strong banana flavour (unless, of course, you prefer that!).

cooking beans from scratch

200g dried beans

8cm piece of kombu (optional)

Fine-grain sea salt or Herbamare, for seasoning *after* cooking

Tip: Be sure not to add salt during the cooking process as it can result in uneven cooking. It's best to season the beans after they cook.

Even though fresh beans always taste superior to canned, I tend to keep canned beans in my pantry for last-minute meals. Eden Organic is a great brand that offers BPA-free cans with kombu added, which aids digestion. Some grocery stores now carry frozen prepared beans, which are so handy – all you have to do is thaw the beans. That said, I do try to prepare beans from scratch whenever possible because the cost savings are huge! On the weekend, soak a pot of beans overnight and cook them up for the week ahead. I like to store leftover beans in the freezer in pre-portioned quantities for quick and easy meals.

Amount varies

PREP TIME: 10 minutes

1. Rinse the beans in a colander.

2. Place the beans in a very large saucepan and add enough water to cover by 8 to 10cm. Soak overnight, or for at least 8 to 12 hours.

3. Drain and rinse the beans thoroughly. Transfer them back to the pan and add fresh water to cover by 5cm. Add the kombu (if using) and stir.

4. Bring the water to the boil over a high heat. With a spoon, skim off the foam and discard. Reduce the heat to medium, and simmer, uncovered, for 30 to 90 minutes (depending on the bean), until the beans are fork-tender and can be easily mashed between your fingers.

5. Drain the beans and season to taste.

6. After cooking a big batch of beans, simply rinse them and allow them to cool. Then refrigerate or freeze any unused beans in containers, jars, or freezer-safe bags, if desired.

roasted garlic

Desired number of garlic heads

Extra-virgin olive oil, for drizzling (optional)

Roasting removes garlic's pungent, sharp bite and leaves behind a sweet, mellow, caramelized buttery flavour that's great on garlic bread, or mixed into pasta sauces, soups, and more. Some people also find it's easier to digest. Once you've tried roasted garlic, you will never see garlic the same way again!

Amount varies

PREP TIME: 5 to 10 minutes • COOK TIME: 35 to 50 minutes

1. Preheat the oven to 200°C (400°F). Peel off the outer layers of skin from the garlic bulb while leaving the skin on the individual cloves.

2. Slice off the top 5mm to 1cm of the head to expose the individual cloves of garlic. If your knife misses a couple of cloves, just use a paring knife to cut the tips off.

3. Set each trimmed garlic head on an individual piece of foil and drizzle with about 1 teaspoon of olive oil, if desired, making sure to cover each exposed clove.

4. Wrap the foil around the garlic and place on a baking sheet or in a muffin tin.

5. Roast for 35 to 50 minutes, until the cloves are golden and soft.

6. Let cool slightly, and then carefully unwrap the garlic bulbs and continue to cool. When the garlic is cool enough to handle, gently squeeze each clove out of its skin and into a bowl. The pungent flavour of raw garlic is now gone, leaving behind a buttery and mild garlic paste.

pumpkin butter

1 to 1.125 litres fresh or canned pure pumpkin puree

60ml sweet apple cider or apple juice, plus more as needed

55g Sucanat or granulated sweetener of choice

3 to 4 tablespoons pure maple syrup, to taste

1 tablespoon ground cinnamon

½ teaspoon freshly grated nutmeg

1 teaspoon pure vanilla extract

1 teaspoon fresh lemon juice

Pinch of fine-grain sea salt

Pumpkin butter epitomizes the fall season, and I make a batch at least once or twice a year. When the blazing orange, red, and yellow leaves start to blanket the great outdoors, I know it's time to pull out this recipe. Smooth, buttery, and velvety, this naturally sweetened pumpkin butter is great served with toast, oatmeal, or parfaits, or simply eaten with a spoon.

Makes about 875ml

PREP TIME: 10 to 30 minutes   •   COOK TIME: 20 to 30 minutes

gluten-free, oil-free, refined sugar-free, nut-free, soy-free, grain-free

1. In a medium-large saucepan, combine the pumpkin, apple cider, sugar, maple syrup, cinnamon, and nutmeg and stir to combine. Cover with the lid and prop the lid ajar with a wooden spoon.

2. Bring the mixture to a low boil over a medium to high heat. Reduce the heat to medium-low and cook, covered, for 20 to 30 minutes, or until thickened. Remove the pan from the heat and let cool for a few minutes. Stir in the vanilla.

3. Let the pumpkin butter cool completely and then stir in the lemon juice and salt. This pumpkin butter will keep in an airtight container in the fridge for 2 to 4 weeks.

Tips: Pumpkin butter is not recommended for canning, but you may be happy to know that it does freeze well and can be kept, frozen, for 1 to 2 months. Thaw at room temperature or in the fridge and stir well before use.

Two (900g) sugar pumpkins should make enough puree for this recipe. To prepare, preheat the oven to 180°C (350°F) and line a very large baking sheet with parchment paper. Slice each pumpkin in half and scoop out all of the seeds. Brush the cut surfaces of the pumpkins with oil and place facedown on the baking sheet.

Roast for 40 to 55 minutes until fork-tender. The exact time will vary based on the size of the pumpkins. Allow to cool, and transfer the flesh to a food processor or blender and process until smooth.

pumpkin pie pecan butter

200g raw pecans, toasted

190g store-bought or homemade pumpkin butter (see page 292)

2 tablespoons pure maple syrup, or to taste

1 teaspoon ground cinnamon

⅛ to ¼ teaspoon freshly grated nutmeg, to taste

¼ teaspoon fine-grain sea salt

1 vanilla bean, scraped (optional)

This is hands-down my favourite spread of all time! That says a lot because I've made a ton of homemade nut butters in my day. Thankfully, homemade pecan butter is a breeze to make. Because pecans have a high oil content and a soft texture, they process into butter in about five minutes. Once you have the pecan butter, simply stir in some pumpkin butter (see page 292) and spices for a spread that will knock your socks off. This Pumpkin Pie Pecan Butter makes a great gift for the holidays – if you can part with it!

Makes 300ml

PREP TIME: 10 minutes

gluten-free, oil-free, soy-free, refined sugar-free, grain-free

1. Preheat the oven to 150°C (300°F). Spread the pecans in a single layer on a rimmed baking sheet and toast them in the oven for 10 to 12 minutes, until fragrant and golden.

2. Process the toasted pecans in a food processor until a butter forms, about 5 minutes, stopping to scrape down the bowl as necessary.

3. Add the pumpkin butter, maple syrup, cinnamon, nutmeg, salt, and vanilla bean seeds (if using) and process until smooth and combined. This spread will keep in an airtight container in the fridge for at least 1 month.

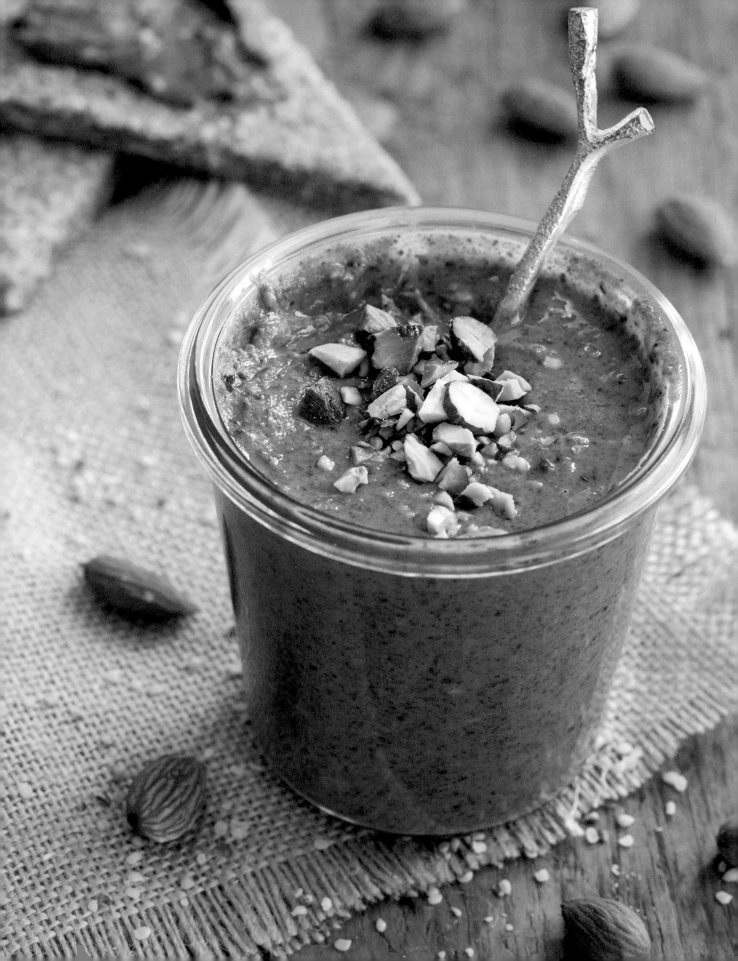

crunchy maple-cinnamon roasted almond butter

315g raw almonds

2 tablespoons pure maple syrup

2 tablespoons hemp seeds

2 tablespoons chia seeds

1 teaspoon ground cinnamon

1 teaspoon pure vanilla extract

1 to 2 teaspoons coconut oil

¼ teaspoon fine-grain sea salt

This almond butter is packed with protein, hemp, and chia seeds, making it a super spread that you can feel good about eating. My advice when making nut butter is to use a heavy-duty food processor – the smaller machines just won't cut it and their motors can burn out.

Makes 300ml

PREP TIME: 20 minutes • COOK TIME: 20 to 25 minutes

gluten-free, soy-free, refined sugar-free, grain-free

1. Preheat the oven to 150°C (300°F). Line a rimmed baking sheet with parchment paper.

2. In a large bowl, combine the almonds and maple syrup and stir to coat the almonds. Spread the almond mixture in a single layer on the prepared baking sheet and bake for 20 to 25 minutes, until fragrant and golden, stirring once halfway through the baking time.

3. Let the almonds cool on the baking sheet for 5 to 10 minutes. If making crunchy almond butter, set aside 35g whole almonds; otherwise, use the entire amount. Process the rest of the almonds in a food processor for 5 to 10 minutes, stopping to scrape the bowl every 30 to 60 seconds as needed.

4. Add the hemp seeds, chia seeds, cinnamon, vanilla, 1 teaspoon of the oil, and the salt. Process until the almond butter is smooth and thin enough to drip off a spoon. Add additional oil if you are having trouble getting the nut butter smooth enough.

5. If making crunchy almond butter, finely chop the reserved almonds and stir them into the almond butter.

6. Store in an airtight glass jar at room temperature or in the fridge for 1 to 2 months.

nutty herb croutons

1 tablespoon ground flaxseed

1 tablespoon extra-virgin olive oil

2 cloves garlic

140g raw almonds

2 tablespoons chopped sweet onion

2 tablespoons packed fresh parsley, or 1 teaspoon dried parsley

2 tablespoons packed fresh basil, or 1 teaspoon dried basil

1 tablespoon fresh thyme, or ½ teaspoon dried thyme

1 tablespoon fresh rosemary, or ½ teaspoon dried rosemary

½ teaspoon dried oregano

¼ teaspoon fine-grain sea salt, or to taste

Herbamare, for sprinkling on top

I promise you will never look at croutons the same way again after trying these nutty, crunchy, flour-free delights. If you are anything like us, you won't be able to stop eating the croutons straight from the pan! Try them with my Chakra Caesar Salad (see page 109) or any salad you wish. See page 111 for a photo.

Serves 8

PREP TIME: 15 minutes • COOK TIME: 30 to 35 minutes
soy-free, sugar-free, grain-free, gluten-free

1. Preheat the oven to 150°C (300°F). Line a large rimmed baking sheet with parchment paper.

2. In a small bowl, combine the flaxseed, oil, and 2 tablespoons of water and stir. Set aside for 5 minutes, stirring occasionally, until the mixture has thickened.

3. In a food processor, pulse the garlic to mince it. Add the almonds and process until finely chopped. Add the onion, parsley, basil, thyme, rosemary, oregano, salt, and flaxseed mixture and process until a sticky ball of dough forms.

4. With your fingers, sprinkle small portions of the crouton dough onto the prepared baking sheet, using roughly ½ teaspoon of dough per crouton. Place the croutons 2.5cm apart on the baking sheet and sprinkle with Herbamare.

5. Bake for 20 minutes, then gently flip the croutons and bake for 10 to 15 minutes more, until golden. Watch the croutons closely near the end of the baking time to make sure they don't burn.

6. Let the croutons cool on the pan for 10 minutes. They will firm up while cooling. Cool the croutons completely and store in an airtight glass jar for 2 to 4 weeks.

balsamic reduction

250ml balsamic vinegar

Vinegar haters need not fear: Once this vinegar cooks down into a syrup, you'll be left with a much sweeter glaze that's lovely drizzled over salads (see my Roasted Beet Salad on page 113), grilled veggies, and seasonal fruit like peaches or strawberries. Or try dipping a fresh baguette into oil and balsamic reduction! That's always a good idea.

It may seem like the recipe calls for a lot of vinegar, but keep in mind that the volume will be reduced by two-thirds by the time we're finished.

Makes about 75ml

PREP TIME: 10 minutes • COOK TIME: 20 to 30 minutes

1. In a medium saucepan, bring the vinegar to a low boil over a medium-high heat. Reduce the heat to medium-low and simmer the vinegar, stirring often, for 20 to 30 minutes, until it has reduced by two-thirds. Keep an eye on the vinegar to avoid burning it and reduce the heat if necessary. You should have about 75ml of reduced balsamic vinegar left in the pan.

2. Remove the pan from the heat and let cool. Transfer the reduction to an airtight container and refrigerate for up to 1 month. The reduction will thicken and firm up once chilled. Allow it to come to room temperature before using.

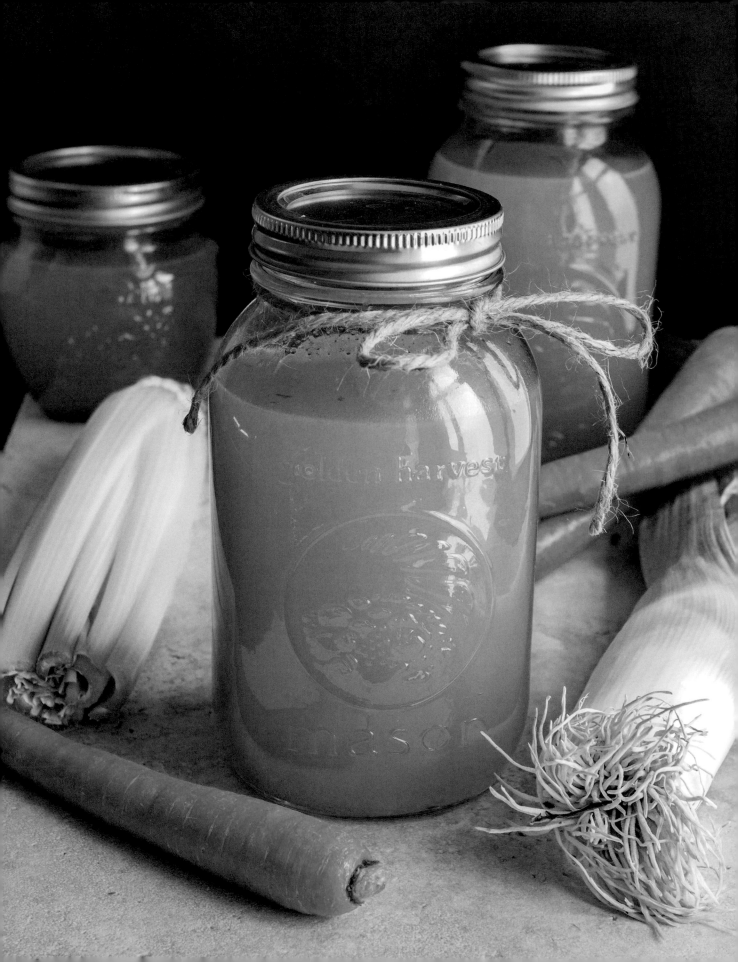

homemade vegetable broth

1½ teaspoons extra-virgin olive oil

3 onions, roughly chopped

1 head garlic, peeled entirely and cloves smashed

Fine-grain sea salt and freshly ground black pepper

3 medium carrots, roughly chopped

4 stalks celery, roughly chopped

1 bunch green onions, roughly chopped

100g shiitake or cremini mushrooms, roughly chopped

1 large tomato, roughly chopped

2 bay leaves

10 sprigs fresh thyme

5cm piece kombu (optional)

1½ teaspoons whole black peppercorns

2 teaspoons fine-grain sea salt

Tip: If you'd like to season the broth even more, add a splash or two of tamari. Keep in mind, however, that it will no longer be soy-free.

For a soy-free option, use coconut aminos.

Making your own broth is certainly not as easy as picking up a few cartons or some bouillon cubes at the grocery store, but there's a true sense of accomplishment when you cook broth from scratch. I like to make a batch at the beginning of 'soup season' so I have it handy. Many store-bought broths contain gluten and yeast, which doesn't work for people with sensitivities, so homemade broth is good to have as an option. I like to freeze this broth in canning jars so they are ready for those chilly, soup-craving winter days. Just be sure to leave a good 2.5cm of space at the top of the jar to allow for expansion. Thanks, America's Test Kitchen, for inspiring this recipe!

Makes 2.4 litres to 2.6 litres
PREP TIME: 30 minutes • COOK TIME: 1½ hours
gluten-free, sugar-free, nut-free, soy-free, grain-free

1. In a large stockpot, heat the oil over a medium heat. Add the onion and garlic and sauté for about 5 minutes. Season with a pinch or two of salt and lots of pepper.

2. Add the carrots, celery, green onions, mushrooms, tomato, bay leaves, thyme, kombu (if using), and peppercorns and sauté for 5 to 10 minutes more.

3. Finally, stir in 2.8 litres water and 2 teaspoons salt. Bring the mixture to a low boil over a high heat. Reduce the heat to medium and simmer for about 90 minutes, or longer if you have the time.

4. Carefully pour the broth through a strainer into a large bowl or pitcher. Compost the solids. Transfer the broth to large glass canning jars, leaving about 2.5cm at the top for expansion. Cool the broth completely, then screw on the lids and place in the freezer. The broth will keep in the freezer for 1 to 2 months or in the fridge for up to 3 days.

5-minute enchilada sauce

2 tablespoons vegan butter or light-tasting oil of choice

2 tablespoons flour

4 teaspoons chilli powder

1 teaspoon garlic powder

1 teaspoon ground cumin

½ teaspoon onion powder

¼ teaspoon cayenne pepper

250ml tomato paste

425ml vegetable broth

¼ to ½ teaspoon fine-grain sea salt, to taste

My homemade enchilada sauce is so finger-licking good, you may never buy store bought again! Use this sauce in my Sweet Potato & Black Bean Enchiladas (see page 147) or simply pair it with a basic dish of greens, beans, and rice.

Makes 500ml

PREP TIME: 5 minutes • COOK TIME: 5 minutes

gluten-free option, nut-free, sugar-free, grain-free

1. In a medium saucepan, melt the vegan butter over a medium heat.

2. Stir in the flour until a thick paste forms. Stir in the chilli powder, garlic powder, cumin, onion powder, and cayenne until combined. Cook for a couple of minutes until fragrant.

3. Stir in the tomato paste, followed by the broth. Whisk until smooth and combined. Bring to a low boil over a high heat (covered, if necessary) and then reduce the heat to medium to maintain a simmer. Stir in salt to taste and simmer for about 5 minutes (or longer, if desired), until thickened.

Tip: For a gluten-free option, use all-purpose gluten-free flour.

basic cooking chart

While this is not intended to be a complete guide to cooking grains or legumes, these are the varieties that I cook with most frequently.

General cooking guidelines for grains: I suggest rinsing grains in a fine-mesh sieve before cooking. This removes debris and prevents unwanted particles from getting into the cooking water. Place the grain and fresh water (or vegetable broth, if desired) in a medium pot and bring to a low boil over a high heat. Reduce the heat to medium-low, cover with a tight-fitting lid, and simmer for the suggested time, or until the grain is tender enough to your liking. Cooking times may differ depending on the heat level and how fresh the grains are, so I suggest keeping an eye on them until you are comfortable with your stovetop. Quinoa, millet, and rice benefit from a five-minute steam after cooking. To do this, simply remove the pan from the heat and let it sit with the lid on for five minutes. Fluff the grains with a fork after steaming.

Last, I added green lentils at the bottom of this chart. Follow the same procedure as above, except simmer the lentils *uncovered* and drain any excess water after cooking.

Please refer to page 290 for instructions on cooking beans.

Grains & Lentils	Dry Amount	Water Amount	Tips	Time	Yield
BASMATI RICE	225g	375ml	Watch closely after 10 minutes.	10 to 15 minutes	600g
GREEN LENTILS	200g	750ml	Simmer lentils uncovered and drain excess water after cooking.	20 to 25 minutes	495g
MILLET	200g	500ml	Lightly toast millet in 1 tablespoon oil before adding water, to enhance flavour.	20 minutes, plus 5 minutes steaming	695g
QUINOA	170g	375ml	Cook with vegetable broth to enhance flavour.	15 to 17 minutes, plus 5 minutes steaming	550g
SHORT-GRAIN BROWN RICE	225g	500ml	Steam for 5 minutes off heat.	40 minutes	550g
SPELT BERRIES	200g	375ml	For chewier spelt berries, reduce cooking time as needed.	35 minutes, or until water is absorbed	400g
WILD RICE	160g	500ml	Steam for 5 minutes off heat.	40 minutes	495g

acknowledgments

They say it takes a village to raise a child and despite my lack of experience with the former, I've been saying these words in regards to creating a cookbook. There are so many talented individuals who poured their hearts into this book and I am so grateful for each and every one of you.

To my husband, Eric, it seems nearly impossible to put into words just how much I love and appreciate you. I've rewritten this paragraph so many times, I've lost count. Selfless, talented, intelligent and pee-your-pants hilarious, you light up my entire life. Throughout my career change, starting the blog and bakery and now this cookbook, you never once cautioned me to take the safer, more predictable path. Thank you for supporting me no matter what crazy venture I set my heart on. The dishes you washed, the grocery lists you checked off and the tears you wiped away are without a doubt why I was able to complete this book. I love you.

I am so grateful for my recipe testers, without whom the recipes in this book wouldn't be nearly as delicious. To my mom, thank you for testing and giving such thorough feedback, as well as sending me recipe clippings for me to 'veganize'. You have always been my biggest cheerleader throughout my life, believing in me when I didn't believe in myself. To my sister Kristi, thank you for testing whenever you could, despite being a busy mother to my amazing nephews. Aunt Diane and Aunt Elizabeth, your generosity with your time and love never ceases to amaze me. Thank you for your support and help with testing. To Tammy Root, for your enthusiasm to test every recipe that I posted and for being upset when it was all over! Finally, a heartfelt thank you to Heather Lutz, Tina Hill, Catherine Bailey, Michelle Bishop, Alyse Nishimura, Donna Forbes, Stefania Moffat, Cindy Yu, Laura Flood and Sara Francoeur.

I am indebted to all of you for giving your time and feedback over the past year! Thank you, thank you, thank you.

To Lucia Watson, my editor at Avery, thank you for your enthusiasm about this project from the beginning and your patience with my intent on getting things just right. We are a great team and I'm so incredibly proud of what we've created. Thanks to Ivy McFadden, for your brilliant copyediting.

Andrea Magyar, my editor at Penguin, thank you for reaching out to me a few years ago and helping me turn my passion into a book. I'm grateful for your constant support, counsel and encouragement throughout this process. Thank you for your diligent work in seeing my vision come to life.

Thanks to my lawyer, James Minns, for helping me slow down and take the time to understand the process. The lessons I've learned through your guidance are invaluable to my career and I'm so grateful to have you by my side. You are a true friend and mentor.

A special thank you to Niki Rockliffe for generously lending us her beautiful kitchen as a backdrop for some of the photography.

To Dave Biesse, it was a real treat to work with you again and have you photograph us playing in the kitchen and outdoors. Thanks for the beautiful images you captured!

To my dear *Oh She Glows* blog readers, I'm in awe of you. Your constant encouragement, support and enthusiasm are without a doubt why I'm here today. Nothing is more exciting than putting your life's passion out into the world and receiving such an encouraging response. You may never know how much I value your comments, questions and feedback, but I truly hope you do. Getting to know you through my blog has made my life richer in so many ways and I hope we'll be able to continue this journey for years to come. I'd love to have the pleasure of meeting more of you in the future!

index

Page numbers in *italics* refer to photos.

about the author

Several years ago, Angela Liddon recovered from an eating disorder, which she battled for more than ten years. Her goal was to learn to love food again while becoming a master in the kitchen. Shortly after earning her master's degree in social psychology and working in the field as a child development researcher, Angela started the blog *Oh She Glows* – a creative outlet where she could write about her journey to health. The response to her writing and recipes was so positive, she soon found herself with thousands of daily readers hungry for more. Eventually she left her career to pursue her passion of blogging, recipe creation and photography full-time. Five years later, *Oh She Glows* has become the destination for healthy vegan recipes around the Web, with millions of page views each month. Her work has been featured in local and international publications such as *VegNews*, *O Magazine*, *Fitness*, *The Kitchn*, *Self*, *Shape*, *National Post*, *The Guardian*, *Glamour* and *Best Health*. *Oh She Glows* has also won several awards, including Veg-News Best Vegan Blog, Chatelaine's Woman of the Year Hot 20 under 30 award and Foodbuzz's Best Veg Blog and Best Overall Blog. When Angela isn't creating recipes or taking pictures of food, she can be found hiking, running, travelling, watching hockey, hanging with girlfriends and embracing her inner yogi. She and her husband, Eric, live in Oakville, Ontario, Canada. Angela's blog can be found online at www.ohsheglows.com.